EXCELLENCE IN NURSING HOMES

Michael A. Patchner, Ph.D., is Professor and Associate Dean at the University of Pittsburgh School of Social Work. He holds a B.A. from California State University of Pennsylvania, a Master of Arts in Sociology and a Master of Social Work from West Virginia University, and a Master of Public Health and a Ph.D. in Social Work from the University of Pittsburgh. Formerly Dean and Professor at West Virginia University, School of Social Work and on the social work faculty at the University of Illinois at Urbana-Champaign, Dr. Patchner has taught courses on social gerontology, health care, social welfare policy, and research. He has 15 years experience consulting with nursing homes and has provided numerous in-service programs for nursing home administrators and staff. Dr. Patchner has administered research projects aimed at improving the quality of care in nursing homes. Most notable is his research on permanently assigning nurses aides to work with residents. He has coauthored two books, *Planning for Research* and *Implementing the Research Plan*, and has published extensively in major social work and health care journals.

Pallassana R. Balgopal, D.S.W., is a Professor in the School of Social Work, University of Illinois at Urbana-Champaign. He also directs the Program for International and Cross-Cultural Social Welfare. He received a B.A. from Nagpur University in India, an M.S.W. from the Madras School of Social Work, a Master of Science in Social Service from Boston University, and a Doctor of Social Work from Tulane University in 1971. Dr. Balgopal combines a broad academic background with extensive experience as a clinical social worker. Prior to joining the University of Illinois faculty in 1978, he taught at the University of Maryland, University of Houston, and Tulane University. He has been a visiting faculty member in India, The Netherlands, and Singapore. He has long been involved in working with individuals, families, and groups, and provides consultation services to professionals within family service agencies, psychiatric settings, and long-term care facilities. Among the texts coauthored by Dr. Balgopal are: *Groups in Social Work: An Ecological Perspective* and *A Three-Dimensional Analysis of Black Leadership*. He has also written numerous journal articles.

EXCELLENCE IN NURSING HOMES

CARE PLANNING, QUALITY ASSURANCE, AND PERSONNEL MANAGEMENT

Michael A. Patchner, Ph.D.
Pallassana R. Balgopal, D.S.W.

Springer Publishing Company
New York

*Dedicated to all the residents
in long-term care facilities*

Copyright ©1993 by Springer Publishing Company, Inc.

All rights reserved.

No part of this publication may be reproduced, stored in a retrieval system, or transmitted in any form or by any means, electronic, mechanical, photocopying, recording, or otherwise, without the prior permission of Springer Publishing Company, Inc.

Springer Publishing Company, Inc.
536 Broadway
New York, NY 10012

93 94 95 96 97 / 5 4 3 2 1

Library of Congress Cataloging-in-Publication Data
Patchner, Michael A.
  Excellence in nursing homes: care planning, quality assurance, and personnel management / Michael A. Patchner, Pallassana R. Balgopal.
    p. cm.
  Includes bibliographical references and index.
  ISBN 0-8261-8150-3
  1. Nursing homes—Administration. 2. Nursing homes—Quality control. 3. Nursing care plans. I. Title.
  [DNLM: 1. Homes for the Aged—organization & administration--United States. 2. Nursing Homes—organization & administration--United States. 3. Patient Care Planning—methods. 4. Personnel Management—methods. 5. Quality Assurance, Health Care—United States. WT 28 AA1 P2e]
RA997.P282   1992
362.1'6'068—dc20
                                                                   92-2217
                                                                     CIP

Printed in the United States of America

CONTENTS

Preface vii

Acknowledgments ix

Part I *Care Planning*

   1 Care Planning Process   3
   2 Assessment   5
   3 Problems, Needs, and Strengths   13
   4 The Care Plan Meeting   19
   5 Goals   29
   6 Approaches   33
   7 Implementation   37
   8 Documentation   43
   9 Evaluation   47
  10 Conclusion   51

Part II *Quality Assurance*

  11 What Is Quality Assurance?   57
  12 Does Quality Assurance Mean Quality Care?   59

13	How Does Quality Assurance Affect Management and Staff?	63
14	How Does Quality Assurance Create a Positive Community Image?	69
15	How Does Quality Assurance Benefit Families?	73
16	How Can Quality Assurance Improve the Nursing Home's Environment?	79
17	Is Quality Assurance Cost Effective?	83
18	Is Quality Assurance Attainable?	87

Part III *Personnel Management*

19	Management Approach	101
20	Staff Composition and Retention	107
21	Advertising and Recruiting	111
22	Hiring	117
23	Personnel Records	125
24	Job Analysis and Job Description	129
25	Salaries and Merit Pay Plan	141
26	Performance Appraisal	147
27	Training and Development	153
28	Staff Morale and Incentive Plans	161
29	Employee Benefits	165
30	Terminations and Layoffs	167

Appendices	*171*
References	*213*
Index	*217*

PREFACE

The variations among nursing homes are as great as the people who live and work in them. Each facility reflects a unique blend of residents and staff whose individual strengths, needs, and values are combined to form the home's own general character and personality. Regardless of the inherent uniqueness of nursing homes, they all share a similar culture. As an interdisciplinary setting, nursing staff, activity workers, physical therapists, physicians, social workers, chaplains, dietitians, housekeepers, and maintenance personnel provide a holistic model of care impacting on the physical, emotional, and spiritual well-being of the residents.

This book examines the nursing home culture and explicates common qualities that yield success. Data for this book were derived from a careful examination of nine facilities in Illinois in addition to a thorough review of the research literature. The nursing homes were selected by the Illinois Department of Public Aid and identified as being exemplary facilities with outstanding reputations for quality service delivery. All research activity and preparation was carried out by the School of Social Work, University of Illinois at Urbana-Champaign. The examination of these facilities revealed three general areas which, when thoroughly developed and strengthened, form a solid foundation for quality service delivery. These three areas have been discussed in a set of previously published separate manuals: *Care Planning Process in Nursing Homes, Quality Assurance in Nursing Homes,* and *Personnel Management in Nursing Homes.*

Each of these topics is now expanded and brought together in one book. The book is divided into three sections which discuss and outline techniques that have proven effective in upgrading service delivery in these facilities. The intent is to provide, under one title, a comprehensive examination of the current nursing home environment by providing fresh and innovative ideas to homes that are struggling as well as to those that have achieved excellence in service delivery.

Part I, *Care Planning*, defines and examines the process for developing care plans which can be effectively used to deliver needed care to the residents and which will maximize their rehabilitative opportunities. A model of step-by-step care planning procedures is offered to be adapted by facilities that are attempting to improve resident care delivery through the care planning process.

Part II, *Quality Assurance*, is a timely examination of what has become one of the most talked about issues in long-term care facilities. This section is intended to define, in concrete and practical terms, the meaning of quality assurance in the nursing home, to describe the benefits of an effective quality assurance program, and to provide guidelines to aid a facility in developing a quality assurance program appropriate to its own unique character and personality. Quality assurance will be examined from a systems perspective. This means that just as quality assurance has a direct effect upon everyone associated with the nursing home, everyone associated with the home has a direct effect upon quality assurance. This duality of people and quality assurance ultimately determines the quality of life for the facility's residents.

Part III, *Personnel Management*, addresses the issue of managing the team of staff, the administrators, owners, and department heads. The issues addressed range from employee morale and turnover to salary programs. The performance appraisal is presented as a key tool for tracking progress and setting goals as well as a tool for providing needed documentation of employee concerns and developing corrective action plans. A list of further readings, which may be helpful in gaining greater depth on a particular subject, is included after all three parts.

The three sections, together, form a holistic approach to providing quality service and resources for the residents, their families, and the community. Improving the quality of service leads to improving the quality of life for nursing home residents, and it is to this end that this book is dedicated.

ACKNOWLEDGMENTS

The writing of this volume involved assistance from many people. Although it is impossible to identify all of them individually, we do want to acknowledge our appreciation to the following individuals and institutions.

We are deeply grateful to the Illinois Department of Public Aid for their interest and the funding that made this research project possible.

Gratitude is also extended to the University of Illinois, School of Social Work for its support. In particular, thanks is expressed to Dean Paula Allen-Meares for her support that helped bring the project to its successful completion.

This project could not have been initiated without the participation and cooperation of the administration and staff of exemplary Illinois nursing homes. Special appreciation is due to the following: Timothy Searby, Administrator, Shirley Ebbersten, DON and John Peterson, Social Service Designee of Christian Nursing Home in Lincoln, Illinois; Marsha Mason, Administrator and Harriet Juliusson, DON of Macomb Nursing and Rehabilitation Center in Macomb, Illinois; Clifford King, Administrator, and Karen Bachman, Social Worker of Maplelawn Home in Eureka, Illinois; Cathy Moses, Past Administrator, Katherine Stanfield, DON and Sherry Bailott, ADON at Americana Healthcare Center of Urbana in Urbana, Illinois; Robert Knobloch, Administrator of Apostolic Christian Home for the Handicapped in Morton, Illinois; Leona Hughes, Administrator, Shirley Stone, Assistant Administrator,

Nancy Finley, DON of Arthur Home in Arthur, Illinois; Jacqueline Mason, Owner, and Joanne Fischer, Administrator of Burgess Square Healthcare Center in Westmont, Illinois; Marsha Reardon, Administrator, and June Bishop, Social Service Designee of Fondulac Manor in Peoria, Illinois; James Bowden, Administrator, Patricia Miller, DON, and Pat Otteney, RN of Lake Bluff Healthcare Center in Lake Bluff, Illinois. We would also like to thank Carol Barkstall, RN, of Parkland Community College, for nursing materials and forms.

Our gratitude is expressed to Jo Schmidt, the Project Director, for her dedication and commitment to this research endeavor. A successful research project cannot be undertaken and completed without a committed and hardworking staff as a foundation. It is our pleasure to commend our project staff for their diligence, insight, and hard work, which contributed very significantly to the success of this project: Debbie J. Barnett, Emer Dean Broadbent, Mary M. Darbes, Debbie Gilpin, Priscilla Purcell, Chathapuram S. Ramanathan, Jerry Ringenberg, Wes Stevens, Becky Witt, and Ronald L. Hastings. Gregory L. Pettys and Gary "Drew" Forrester need to be recognized for their assistance in the final revision of this volume.

Finally, our wives, Lisa Patchner and Shyamala Balgopal, and our children, Christopher and Maria, and Meena and Anita, deserve very special thanks for their caring and love, without which this volume would not have become a reality.

PART I

CARE PLANNING

INTRODUCTION

The authors initially had mixed feelings about the care planning process, feelings which originated from their experiences as nurses aides, nurses, social workers, social work consultants, and long-term care researchers. After conducting research in long-term care facilities, the authors arrived at the following conclusions: first, care planning makes a difference; second, effective care planning is possible.

In the literature, considerable information is found concerning how to write nursing care plans in hospital settings and how individual departments should write assessments and evaluations. However, very little is found on how departments in nursing homes should do care planning. Part I begins to fill the "how to" gap in this area.

The section is organized for use in nursing homes by nursing home staff, regardless of level of experience. The inexperienced worker as well as the seasoned care delivery expert will benefit from the concepts, organizational suggestions, text, examples, sample forms, and checklists.

Part I begins with a brief overall view of the continuous nursing home care planning process. Special attention is given to the care plan document itself. After this familiarization chapter, the text follows the care plan process step by step from beginning to end as follows: Assessment, Problems/Needs, Care Plan Meetings, Goals, Approaches, Implementation, Documentation, and Evaluation.

Appendices are included to give care planners ideas of what information to include in resident assessment and other forms, and ideas of how they can construct forms that meet their own facility's and residents' needs.

This section is by no means intended to address all care planning problems faced by facility staff. The intent is to give the facility staff tools to address their own respective problems.

Chapter 1

CARE PLANNING PROCESS

All long-term care facilities develop care plans for their residents. The purpose of care planning is to provide the best possible care for each resident; care which will address each resident's specific needs and maximize his or her rehabilitative potential. The care planning process involves systematic, coordinated, and planned procedures for development and delivery of necessary care. Successful care planning can be of great benefit to all nursing home residents and staff.

The care planning process is often seen as being quite complicated. However, the process can be more easily understood by examining the following steps, which are essential for effective care planning to occur.

1. Assess the resident's physical and psychosocial condition to identify the resident's problems, needs, and strengths.
2. Hold interdisciplinary meetings to formulate a care plan for each resident. During the meeting state the problems and develop goals and approaches related to each problem.
3. Implement the care plan.
4. Document the delivery of care.
5. Evaluate the effectiveness of the approaches and goals.
6. After a given time, revise the care plan and repeat steps 1–5. (See Figure 1.1)

An interdisciplinary team effort underlies the entire care plan process. Team principles that support the care plan process are coopera-

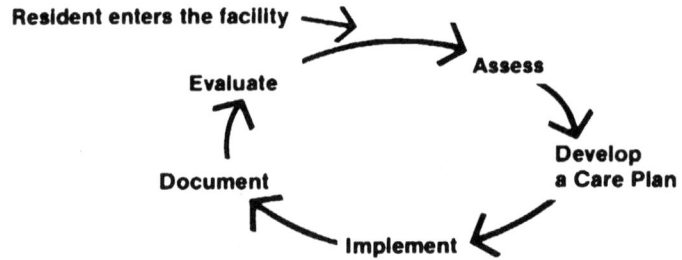

FIGURE 1.1 The care planning process.

tion, discussion, consensus, shared responsibility, and coordination. These principles, which are evident throughout the process, take on an extra significance during the care plan meeting.

The interdisciplinary team effort is the essential dynamic of care plan meetings. Care plan team members combine their professional experience and expertise during the discussion on problems, needs, and strengths, and during the development of goals and approaches. The outcome of this team meeting is a care plan which reflects the combined input of all facility staff via the team members.

The coordination of services is outlined by the care plan. The care plan functions very simply as a map for staff to follow as they interact with and deliver care to residents. By looking at the care plan, the care planning process becomes apparent. The care plan form contains the following areas:

Resident Problems, Needs, and Strengths—descriptions of the resident's conditions which receive staff attention.

Resident Goals—the specific statements which measure staff effectiveness in alleviating resident needs.

Staff Approaches—the strategies to be employed for attaining resident goals.

Responsibility—the person or department assigned to implement the approach.

The care planning process focuses on these areas of the care plan in order to provide effective care services in the most efficient manner. (An example of care plan development from diagnosis to approach is outlined in Appendix K.)

Chapter 2

ASSESSMENT

The assessment step in the care planning process provides the foundation on which care is based. The purpose of assessment is for the staff to gain familiarity and understanding of the resident and family so that a cooperative relationship can be established to provide quality care. Concerning the care planning process, the outcome of assessment is the identification of problems, needs, and strengths.

A detailed description of each resident emerges from a composite of the assessments made by representatives from each therapeutic area of the facility including nursing, activities, social services, dietary, rehabilitation services, and others. Assessment can be compared to a situation where a person wants to get a complete idea of what a statue looks like. This person has photographs taken from many different positions around the statue. Each photo is of the same subject, but presents a different view of it. Each picture contributes to a complete understanding and appreciation of what the statue looks like. During resident assessment, many departmental "photographers" take "pictures" of the resident through their own particular profession's "camera." Nursing creates a nursing assessment, social services takes a social history, and so forth through dietary, rehabilitation, activities, and others.

A complete description of the resident emerges from a composite of observations made by representatives from each professional department in the facility (see Figure 2.1). Each view of the resident is important, and when all are combined, a complete understanding of the resident is established, allowing decisions to be

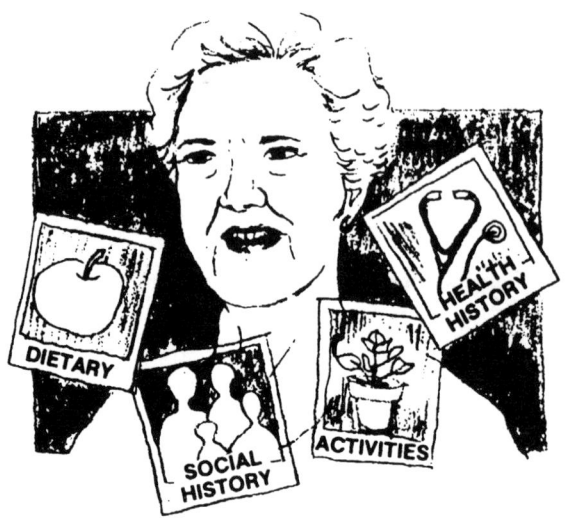

FIGURE 2.1 Combining professional assessments gives a comprehensive picture of the resident.

made on effective treatment. This composite view is not only carried out at admission to the facility, but occurs continuously over time as a method of marking progress in resident treatment and as a basis for revising care plans.

Assessment benefits the resident, the facility, and the staff by assuring that:

- The resident receives care which addresses actual needs.
- The resident receives care which eliminates relevant problems.
- The facility appropriately and effectively treats resident problems.
- Staff morale improves because staff sees positive results from effective care delivery.

The following is an example of the importance of assessment:

> Mr. X arrived in the facility three days ago from the hospital. He is confused and somewhat combative. Each department did an initial assessment and the care plan meeting is in progress. During the discussion of initial assessment interviews and goals, the head of activities, who

has a comprehensive information collecting system, asks the nursing representative, "Will the resident's scabies interfere with his participation in activity programs?" The nurse responds with surprise because she was not aware of this condition.

In this facility, only the activities representative, from careful examination of the resident and of hospital discharge papers, noticed and considered a very important piece of admission data about Mr X. Without this information the care plan team would have developed a care plan based upon an incomplete picture of the resident. Such a lack could have proven dangerous to the resident, other residents, and staff.

In the next section the steps for assessment of a resident are detailed—steps that the facility in the above example should have followed.

Steps of assessment are:

1. Learn about a resident before admission.
2. Inform each department of a new resident.
3. Assign responsibility for the assessment.
4. Collect information.
5. Identify problems, needs, and strengths.
6. Continue ongoing assessment.
7. Perform reassessment periodically.

LEARN ABOUT THE RESIDENT BEFORE ADMISSION

Admissions personnel begin assessment before the resident enters the facility. They gather information from the preadmission screening and doctor's exam to give the facility staff a general idea of the resident's problems. This information is discussed among staff members informally (e.g., conversations in the halls) or formally (e.g., during administrative or other staff meetings).

The admissions process will vary from facility to facility, but should contain the following steps:

1. An inquiry for admission is received from the prospective resident, the resident's family, or the hospital.

2. A home or hospital visit is made by a facility representative. Information may also be obtained from telephone conversations and family/resident visits to the facility.
3. The person's major diagnoses, problems, needs and strengths are identified by studying the doctor's reports and by contacting the resident, family, hospital social worker or nurse.
4. Information is shared among appropriate staff and a decision to admit the person is made.

INFORM EACH DEPARTMENT OF A NEW RESIDENT

Collect introductory resident information that is important to the facility and record it on a form. (See Appendix A.) Distribute introductory resident information to each department. This information announces the admission of a new resident.

ASSIGN RESPONSIBILITY FOR THE ASSESSMENT

Assign one person within each department to perform initial departmental assessments. The benefits of designating a specific person to do the assessments are:

- There is an increased likelihood of having a timely initial assessment because assessment responsibility is clearly assigned.
- The care plan team will know whom to contact if they have questions about the assessment.
- The language used in assessments will be consistent from resident to resident, allowing the care plan team and care delivery staff to know what is meant by what is written.

Assessment 9

COLLECT INFORMATION

Follow established procedures for performing the initial assessment with each resident. Diagnoses, descriptions, and other elements of the assessment will be equally and predictably complete, accurate, and understandable for each resident who enters the facility. Consistency of procedure, writing format, language and technique will provide a clear understanding of the resident's needs:

- Each department transfers preliminary information onto their respective assessment forms, which act as tools for gathering resident data. The assessment form, whether it is in a checklist, narrative, or other format, reminds staff of the information they need to obtain and allows for the recording of this information.
- Each department creates its own assessment forms by incorporating certain generally accepted areas of assessment information into the form and by including other areas that are uniquely important to the facility, the department, and resident population. The format, too, can be tailored to meet the specific needs of the staff that will be using the forms. Checklists of suggested assessment information items and examples of assessment forms that may be used by the different departments can be found in Appendices B through E.

Information about residents is collected through observations, interviews, and an examination of documents. The following sources of information can be used for assessment data:

- Resident
- Resident's family and friends
- Facility staff
- Documentation
- Community agency personnel
- Physicians and hospital personnel

Use a comprehensive form for assessment and consistent, simple language. Use words that are simple enough to be understood by all staff. Beware of the use of technical terms. For example, use a nursing diagnosis in place of a medical diagnosis: "shortness of breath" instead of "emphysema." In addition, it is better not to use abbreviations unless all staff know what they mean. In the above example "shortness of breath" is often written as "S.O.B." Unless all staff are aware of this abbreviation, they may think that it stands for something else.

IDENTIFY PROBLEMS, NEEDS, AND STRENGTHS

The department head or departmental care plan team member uses the information to identify problems, needs, and strengths. These problems, needs, and strengths will be discussed at the care plan meeting.

CONTINUE ONGOING ASSESSMENT

Care delivery must be responsive to changes in the resident's condition. Continue to collect assessment data so staff can identify a resident's changing physical and psychological health. Note changes in the nature of the resident's problems and needs. If the resident's condition changes unexpectedly, then propose a care plan revision.

PERFORM REASSESSMENT PERIODICALLY

Formal periodic reassessments precede care plan reviews which occur every 60 days for skilled care residents, every 90 days for intermediate care residents, or within 14 days following a significant change in a resident's status. These reassessments prepare staff for the next care plan meeting by identifying progress on previous goals, changes in health, and by identifying current problem and needs.

THE RESIDENT ASSESSMENT INSTRUMENT AND MINIMUM DATA SET

Medicare and Medicaid approved facilities are required to conduct comprehensive, accurate, standardized, and reproducible assessments of each resident's functioning capacity using a Resident Assessment Instrument (RAI) which is specified by the state. At a minimum each state's RAI must include the Minimum Data Set (MDS), which is a requirement of the federal government's Health Care Financing Administration.

In itself, the MDS provides information about each resident, including a minimum core of assessment items, with definitions and coding categories needed to make a more comprehensive assessment. Areas for assessment with the MDS are:

- identifying and background information
- cognitive patterns
- vision patterns
- physical functioning and structural problems
- continence in the past 14 days
- psychosocial well-being
- mood and behavior patterns
- activity pursuit patterns
- disease diagnosis
- health conditions
- oral/nutritional status
- oral/dental status
- skin condition
- medication use
- special treatments and procedures

While the MDS is most often completed by various health professionals assessing their specialty area, the RN coordinator is responsible for completing the MDS or coordinating its completion with the appropriate participation of other health professionals. At least one MDS assessment and three quarterly reviews in each 12-month period will be done for each resident to ensure that care plans are meeting current needs. Additional MDS assessments are completed within a 14-day period following a significant change in residence status.

The MDS is used for preliminary assessment and screening of resident problems. From the MDS key characteristics of a resident's problems can be identified and "triggers," which alert the assessor to the resident's potential problems or needs, can identify conditions necessary to consider in making care plan decisions. For example, if a resident is identified from the MDS as being incontinent two or more times a week or uses catheters or pads, then this automatically "triggers" a care plan need for improving urinary continence.

Chapter 3

PROBLEMS, NEEDS, AND STRENGTHS

Typically, problems and needs are thought of as a single unit (problems/needs) by nursing home personnel. For the purposes of explanation, this text will address them individually and introduce the role of strengths.

Problems are any physiological or psychosocial conditions which prevent the resident from fulfilling his or her needs, threaten the resident's personal well-being, or reduce the resident's quality of life.

Needs are physiological or psychosocial requirements that must be met by or for the resident to achieve or maintain his or her well-being or quality of life. Residents have needs that must be fulfilled.

Strengths are areas of resident proficiency, physiological, or psychosocial assets, that can be used by the resident or staff to fulfill a need.

The aging process presents often irreversible problems to residents. These problems prevent a resident from independently fulfilling his or her own needs. Resident problems, needs, and strengths are identified in the assessment step of the care planning process. Resident needs come to the attention of the facility during assessment when it becomes apparent that problems prevent their fulfillment. It is the task of the nursing home to mobilize its resources and those of the resident (e.g., resident strengths) in an effort to eliminate or reduce the impact of problems on resident need fulfillment.

When considering problems, needs, and strengths, follow these steps:

1. Identify resident's problems and needs.
2. Identify resident's strengths.
3. Present the problems, needs, and strengths at the care plan meeting.

IDENTIFY A RESIDENT'S PROBLEMS AND NEEDS

During assessment, identify specific conditions (problems) that negatively affect the resident's lifestyle, needs fulfillment, and quality of life. Record these problems (with their accompanying needs written in, or implicit) on the assessment form and develop a problem list.

There are four major categories of problems. Implicit corresponding needs are also offered in the examples.

Diagnosis-Linked Problems

List the resident's diagnoses, problems associated with each diagnosis, and the needs with which the problems interfere. The diagnosis is not the problem. Attention is focused on the symptoms or behaviors which are associated with the diagnosis that impede resident functioning. For example:

diagnosis	osteo-arthritis
problem	joint pain
need	(A need is for the resident to be) free from joint pain

Medical or Functional Problems

List any problematic medical or functional conditions that are unrelated to a diagnosis. Identify the problem's results or effects on fulfillment of the resident's needs. For example:

problems	high potential for skin breakdown/wet clothing/urinary incontinence
need	(The resident has a need for) healthy skin

Psychosocial Problems

List emotional, mental, social, and behavioral problems and their effects on the resident's functioning. For example:

problems	disorientation/unable to find room/fails to recognize family members/arrives late for meals
needs	(The resident has a need to) be safe/be able to find own room/socialize/eat

Management Problems

List resident traits, behaviors, characteristics, or idiosyncrasies which are problematic and require staff awareness and management in order to ensure fulfillment of needs.

problems	refuses to accept medication/dumps lunch plate onto the floor
needs	(A need exists for the resident to) take medication/maintain weight at present level

Maslow's hierarchy of needs identifies five levels of needs which address healthy personality development. This hierarchy can be adapted to resident's needs fulfillment and personality development. Need fulfillment is relevant as a resident copes with and adjusts to the nursing home environment and his/her changing physical and psychosocial condition. Consider these development areas when discussing resident needs in the nursing home context and prioritize the needs by using the following list. Basic and safety needs must be met before moving on to higher order needs. There are:

- Basic needs such as food, or freedom from pain
- Safety and security needs such as feelings of trust towards staff

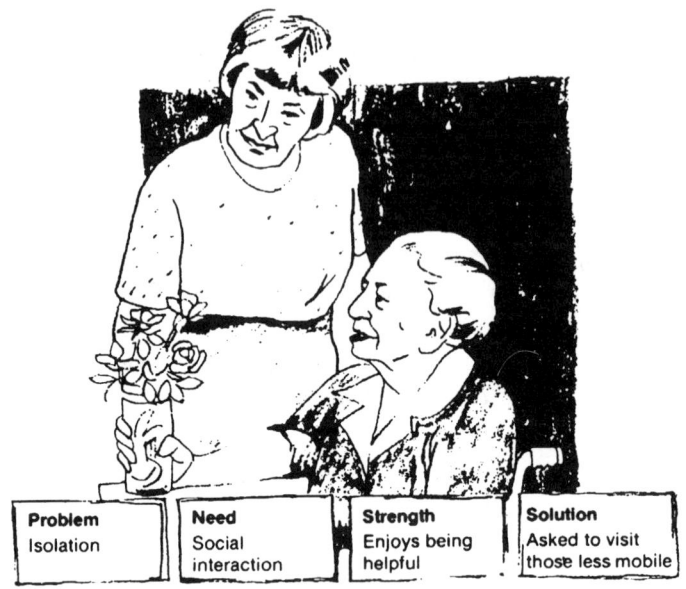

FIGURE 3.1 Use resident strengths to address problems and to meet needs.

- Belonging and love needs such as being an active participant in family relationships
- Social esteem and self respect needs such as being president of Resident Council
- Self-actualization needs such as being at peace with oneself.

IDENTIFY A RESIDENT'S STRENGTHS

During assessment, develop a picture of the whole person by identifying areas of resident proficiency or strengths. These abilities may be used as resources during implementation of the care plan to counteract the effects of problems on resident needs. (See Figure 3.1.) Use of resident strengths is an empowering way to involve the resident in personal care delivery and is likely to increase the achievement rate of the care plan goals.

Examples of resident strengths include:

- Food likes
- Musical or verbal talents
- Supportive family
- Excellent walking skills
- Enjoys socializing
- Aptitude for craft work.

Strengths may be incorporated into the problems/needs section on the care plan form in the following way so that effective approaches can be developed to achieve resident goals:

problem	weight loss
need	(a need for the resident is to) maintain a stable weight
strength	resident loves Bohemian cooking
diagnosis	terminal cancer of the colon
problem	grief
need	(a need exists for the resident to) come to terms with life experiences and accept the consequences of the diagnosis
strength	supportive family members.

PRESENT THE PROBLEMS, NEEDS, AND STRENGTHS

Discuss resident's identified problems, needs, and strengths during the care plan meeting. Be prepared to consider the following points during the discussion:

- Chances of effective intervention
- Degree of threat to the resident's health
- Potential benefits for the resident.

Chapter 4

THE CARE PLAN MEETING

The care plan meeting is the formal gathering of staff to formulate a resident's care plan. It is during this meeting that systematic planning of care is openly discussed to produce a written care plan that coordinates services provided to a resident. Representatives from all the facility's departments attend this meeting. This creates an interdisciplinary setting that includes nursing, dietary, activities, housekeeping, social services, rehabilitation services, and staff from other relevant departments. In addition, the resident and the resident's family are invited to attend the meeting (see Figure 4.1).

Conduct a care plan meeting by following these steps:

1. Create a productive setting
2. Develop a meeting schedule
3. Select an interdisciplinary team
4. Involve residents and family members
5. Designate a coordinator
6. Delegate duties among team members
7. Evaluate goals
8. Discuss the resident's problems, needs, and strengths
9. Develop the care plan
10. Record information on the care plan form
11. Communicate the care plan to direct care providers
12. Repeat the previous five steps (7–11)
13. Adjourn.

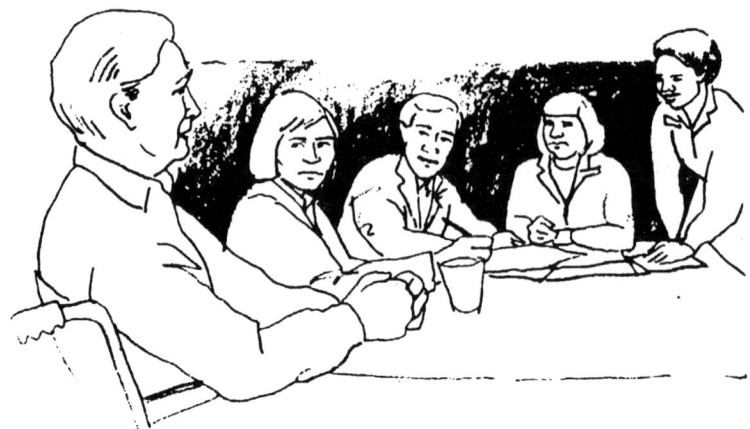

FIGURE 4.1 Resident is included in the care planning process.

Create a Productive Setting

The physical setting in which the meeting occurs impacts on the operation of the meeting and the formulation of the care plan.

Consider the following points when structuring the physical setting of the meeting.

- Select a quiet, private room for the meeting. Privacy is crucial for the team to have open discussions about the residents.
- Use a table large enough to seat all team members and to hold all charts and paperwork. Team members must feel comfortable and have necessary workspace.
- Hold the meeting at a convenient time for attendance so the members will be able to contribute quality participation and input.
- Do not allow distractions or interruptions during the meeting. Inform the receptionist to take phone messages for team members. The focus of attention during the meeting should be on the development of the resident's care plan.
- Provide beverages and/or snacks. Refreshments create a relaxed atmosphere in which to work.

The setting strongly affects the quality of input that team members offer during meetings. To ensure an input-intensive setting remember to:

- Respect others' input. Avoid personally critical statements. Offer constructive commentary that contributes to the care plan.
- Encourage professional interaction among staff to build team spirit. This promotes professional trust rather than personal distrust.
- Carefully choose the care plan coordinator. Designate a person who sparks focused discussion among members.

Develop a Meeting Schedule

The tremendous flow of care plans warrants attention to scheduling and processing. A care plan must be developed shortly after admission for all newly admitted and readmitted residents. For intermediate care residents, the care plan must be revised at least every 90 days and for skilled care residents, at least every 60 days. As previously unidentified problems and needs emerge, "between period" revisions will also be scheduled.

Scheduling depends upon:

- Number and care level of residents in the facility
- Amount of time spent on each care plan
- Frequency of meetings
- Length of meetings
- Number of care plans completed in each meeting.

These scheduling factors affect the flow and processing of the care plans. The care plan coordinator needs to determine how often to meet and for how long (frequency and length of meetings). Staff must be informed of the frequency and duration of meetings in order to make preparations and to reserve necessary time.

The number of residents, level of care, and the average amount of time spent for each care plan determine the total amount of time required for care plan meetings. Remember to plan time for hospital readmissions and between period revisions.

Example: Loving Care Nursing Home has 100 residents living at the intermediate care level. According to the regulations each resident's care plan must be revised every 90 days (a period of 12 weeks). This means that between eight or nine care plans must be completed weekly.

Including hospital readmissions, which occur randomly, a conservative schedule would plan for ten care plans per week. If the team averages about half an hour per resident, then 5 hours must be allocated for the care plan meetings each week. Loving Care Nursing Home decides how often and when to meet based upon the 5 average hours per week. For example, the home may decide to meet 5 days per week for about an hour or may meet 3 days per week or every other day for a little over 1 and 1/2 hours.

- 100 residents divided by 12 weeks (90 days) equals eight or nine cases weekly, and hospital readmissions increase weekly cases to ten.
- Ten cases multiplied by 1/2 hour per case equals 5 hours per week for care plan meetings

Things to consider when deciding how often and how long to hold meetings include the following:

- Keep the length of the meeting short. Members will remain attentive and maintain efficiency during the meeting.
- Schedule meetings several times per week. This builds a routine for members and enhances effectiveness.
- Be flexible when conditions require additional meetings or longer meetings. A sudden influx of new residents, hospital readmissions, or between period revisions will place demands on the usual schedule.

Scheduling helps assure that all care plans are completed on time. Having a schedule also allows the care plan team to prepare for the meetings. The care plan coordinator, therefore, must:

- Prepare a monthly or weekly schedule of care plans and distribute to team members ahead of time. With a schedule of upcoming care plans, team members can make preparations for the meeting.
- Prepare a yearly calendar of care plans. Scheduling care plan revisions prevents overlooking or forgetting that a residents' plan is due for review. To prepare a yearly schedule, use a calendar or divide a notebook into months by designating a page for each month. When a resident is admitted to the facility, schedule the initial care plan meeting and tentatively record the resident's name on the schedule book every 90 days

(for intermediate care residents) or every 60 days (for skilled care residents). Allot some days or time for hospital readmissions and betwteen period revisions.

Select an Interdisciplinary Team

Care plan meetings must be interdisciplinary, which means that representatives from all departments in the facility participate in the meeting. Attendance at a care plan meeting should include, but not be limited to a nurse (DON and/or charge nurse), the social service designee, rehabilitative staff (e.g., nurse, physical therapist, occupational therapist, speech therapist, or their aides), activity director, dietary director, and whenever possible, the resident and/or family member.

The staff present at the meeting may vary from resident to resident. Often, other personnel are called into the meeting to offer information about a resident. For example a nurse's aide, housekeeper, an activity aide, administrator, pharmacist, physician, or consultants (e.g., social worker, dietary, etc.).

Team members who formulate statements, goals, and approaches on the care plan are often department heads. They must be knowledgeable about how to use the resources of the facility, the staff, and the residents.

Involve Residents and Family Members

Resident and family involvement benefits the care planning process. Involvement helps residents and families emerge as care delivery resources. For example, the family members may be involved by taking the resident on weekly community outings, reading letters, or providing personal grooming tasks.

The involvement process is unique to every home. Involvement at the care plan meeting can be facilitated by inviting residents and family members to meetings to give their input to the care planning process. To encourage resident and family involvement:

- Send letters, make telephone calls, or personally invite residents and their families to the meeting in advance. Explain

the reasons for the care plan meeting and stress the value of the person's input.
- Welcome the resident and family to the meeting. Make introductions to everyone in the room.
- Review the care plan with the resident and family. Pause frequently to ask for input, suggestions, or comments.
- Listen to the remarks of the resident and family. Offer explanations when necessary.
- Incorporate the resident's and family's suggestions into the care plan.

Designate a Coordinator

The care plan coordinator is given the role of meeting leader. The main responsibility of this position is to ensure the development of the care plan and to plan the schedule. A care plan coordinator may be chosen from any profession. Characteristically, an effective coordinator:

- Exhibits leadership skills, e.g., motivates the team to get the job done
- Facilitates open discussion and input from all team members
- Communicates proficiently, both verbally and in writing.

Delegate Duties Among Team Members

The coordinator of the care plan meeting may assume one of various styles of leadership, which exerts considerable influence on team members' performance of their duties. Two common styles are "shared leadership" and "singular leadership" (see Table 4.1).

Shared leadership occurs when the care plan coordinator delegates duties and tasks among the several team members. For example, the coordinator may have the activity representative gather assessment data from all departments on a particular resident before the meeting occurs, and have the representative take charge of the care plan meeting during discussion of that resident. This allows division of the caseload among staff and promotes staff investment in the resident's care plan.

TABLE 4.1 Comparison of Leadership Styles for Care Planning Team

Issues	Shared leadership	Singular leadership
Responsibility/ accountability for duties	Duties of the meeting are divided among team members. Leadership roles shift between members.	The leader performs most of the meeting duties. Everyone knows who leads.
Communication patterns	Information flows between team members.	Information flows through the singular leader.
Staying on schedule	Workload is shifted between members to stay on schedule.	Mainly relies on attendance and productivity of leader.
Team spirit	Sharing duties among members builds a sense of competence.	Team spirit is maintained by the leader.
Level of success	Depends on the interaction and input from all team members.	Depends on the leader's abilities.

In singular leadership most of the tasks and duties of care plan development are performed by the coordinator. Collection of evaluation data, preparations of tentative problem and needs statements and goals, and scheduling of revisions are all performed by the coordinator who uses this style. To be successful, this form of leadership requires a coordinator who is fast-acting, determined, and highly energetic.

Evaluate Goals

Before new goals are discussed, evaluate previous goal achievement. To aid in decision-making, utilize several sources of information.

- Utilize documentation, staff, resident, and family.
- Use the information to help determine if the resident met the goal.

- For goals that have not been achieved, determine if the goal is:
  —attainable in its present form and should be carried over to the next care plan period,
  or
  —unattainable in its present form and should be altered before being carried over to the next care plan period,
  or
  —unattainable and should be abandoned.
- For goals that have been achieved, determine if the continued existence of resident problems and needs warrants creation of a new goal to address the same problems and needs.

Discuss the Resident's Problems, Needs, and Strengths

- Discuss the problems, needs, and strengths that were identified during assessment.
- Discuss the effects of each problem and need on the resident's well-being and determine the degree of threat to the resident's health.
- Consider the resources of the facility and strengths of the resident which counteract the problems and needs.
- Decide which problems, needs, and strengths to include on the care plan by matching problems and needs to available resources. Seek to minimize threats to the resident's well-being.

Develop the Care Plan

For each problem and need goals are established and a series of approaches is developed to facilitate meeting of the goals by the resident.

- Use information from the previous goals to help establish:
  —Which goals were achieved
  —Whether the goal solved the problem and fulfilled the need
  —Which approaches were effective
  —What are current resident performance levels
  —What are potential resident performance levels.

- Ask and consider what each department can do to alleviate the problem and fulfill the need using the resources available to them.
    1. Decide on new or additional approaches.
    2. Decide on new or additional goals.
- Use information from past and current decision-making to select new approaches and goals.
- Assign responsibility for each approach (e.g., designate the persons or departments that are responsible for each treatment approach).

Record Information on the Care Plan Form

Record problems, needs, strengths, goals, approaches, and responsible entities on the care plan form.

- Use simple language so everyone who reads the care plan can understand it.
- Write neatly so the reader can understand the care plan.
- Write in ink.
- Establish a code for communicating goal achievement status (e.g., marking a goal with a yellow highlighter indicates goal achievement and discontinuation of that goal).

Develop a care plan form that reflects the unique needs and characteristics of the facility, the staff, and the resident. Consider several concepts and characteristics for inclusion:

- Use simple, clearly worded headings for each section to assist personnel who write and read the care plan document.
- Provide generous amounts of space for the writing of the statement of problems, needs, goals, and approaches.
- Communicate the care plan to care givers. Keep previous care plans so a history or progression is accessible to staff. Add pages when the current form is full.

(See Appendices F, G, and H for ideas on contents of care plan and format of care plan form.)

Communicate the Care Plan to Direct Care Providers

- Write the new care plan information on communication forms used by direct care providers, e.g., care cards and goal checklists. (See Appendices I and J.)
- Update the care plan communication forms during the care plan meeting.
- Record approaches, goals, and responsibilities on communication forms.
- Use simple language and abbreviations that are under-standable to everyone.

Repeat the Five Previous Steps

For each resident's care plan repeat the following steps:

- Evaluate goals.
- Discuss the resident's problems, needs, and strengths.
- Develop the care plan.
- Record information on the care plan form.
- Communicate the care plan to the direct care providers.

Adjourn

End the meeting when all scheduled residents' care plans are completed.

Chapter 5

GOALS

Goals are specific, resident-centered action statements which measure a resident's progress towards problem resolution and need fulfillment. Goals are measurement tools as well as statements of accomplishment. To develop effective goals, the care plan team must:

1. Develop resident goals.
2. Keep diagnoses and discharge potential in mind.
3. State goals in realistic, behavioral, and measurable terms.

DEVELOP RESIDENT GOALS

Interdisciplinary discussion during the care plan meeting results in better development of goals. Team members share their creative and technical ideas for each resident's goal. Team discussion of goals builds support for care plan implementation.

A reasonable relationship must exist between the goal and the identified problem and need. Goals must be behaviorally related to the resident's problem and need (e.g., resident will walk 25 feet, resident will go to three activities per week, etc., see Figure 5.1). Progress towards the goal signifies a step towards solving a problem or alleviating the resident's need.

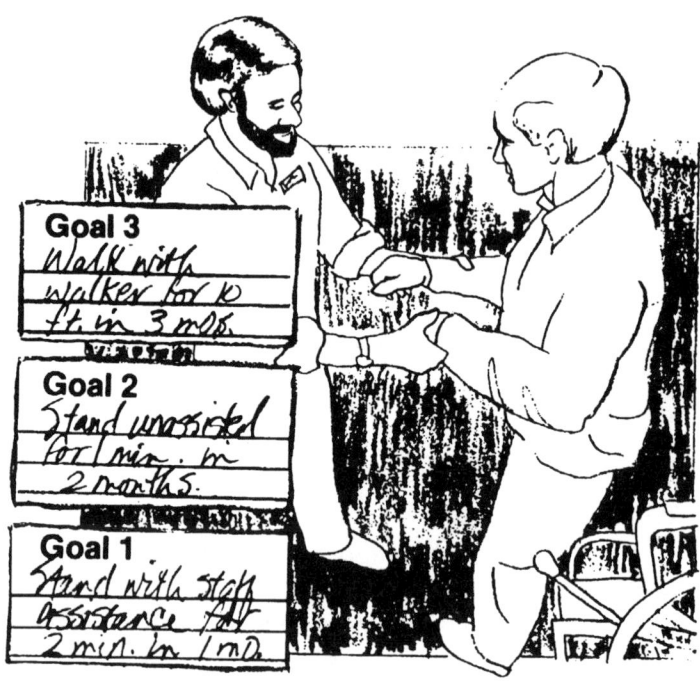

FIGURE 5.1 Goals reflect resident progress.

KEEP DIAGNOSES AND DISCHARGE POTENTIAL IN MIND

Staff need to have a far-sighted, future view of a resident's potential mental and physical health. This future view is based upon the resident's strengths and capacity to improve. There are three categories of resident care outcomes:

Rehabilitation—The resident has a chance to return to the community.

Institutionalization—The resident will live in the nursing home for an indefinite period of time.

Terminal care institutionalization—The resident faces imminent death.

Careful assessment and experience in geriatric health care provide a basis to foresee a resident's probable outcome.

STATE GOALS IN REALISTIC, BEHAVIORAL, AND MEASURABLE TERMS

Goals are developed to challenge the resident and stimulate improvements in his/her quality of life. There are many areas and types of goals (see Appendix H). Goals should be:

Concise—Avoid unnecessary words and repetition

Resident-centered—The resident is the subject of the statement. The goal describes an action of the resident or a change in the resident's condition.
  Example:
  - (The resident will) "walk 25 feet per day independently with a walker."
  - (The resident's) "decubitus reduced to 1 cm by (date)."

Action oriented—A resident's response is stated in observable or tangible terms. Begin each statement with an action verb, to alert the staff to the precise resident behavior to be observed upon goal achievement.
  Examples:

Speak	Wash	Cough	Reduce
Walk	Eat	Stop	Demonstrate
Transfer	Drink	Hold	Give
Identify	Sleep	Read	Decrease

Specific—Describe exactly what is expected to occur. The content is the object of the action verb. It identifies the area of change in the patient's condition or behavior that should be observable when the goal is achieved.

Measurable—Use phrases that describe concrete, objective, measurable occurrences; amounts, numbers, distances, timespan, test results, facts, etc. Avoid phrases that require subjective judgement or getting a general impression. Identify times, place, person.
  Example:
  Walk 25 feet. Transfer from bed to chair. Wash self. Eat chopped foods. Drink two pitchers of water every day.

Precise—Add modifying words or phrases to define the content area as precisely as possible. Modifiers answer questions such as when, where, how, how much, how far, with what help, with whose help, etc.

Example:
Walk 25 feet independently with walker. Transfer from bed to chair with supervision. Wash self with assistance of one person.

Clear—Words like "better, worse, good, bad, more, less," even "depression and agitation," require further qualification. They can mean different things to different people.

Understandable—Make certain everyone concerned knows all the terms, abbreviations, codes and symbols used.

Realistic—Goal achievement requires effort from the resident but is within his/her capabilities to attain.

Time limited—Evaluation of the goal occurs at a specific date.

Chapter 6

APPROACHES

Approaches state what staff and family will do to help the resident achieve care plan goals. Approaches tell staff "what to do" and "how to do it" for the resident. Use of the suggested approaches listed in the care plan increases the likelihood that the resident will achieve his or her care plan goal. Follow these steps:

1. Develop approaches.
2. List the approaches.
3. Assign responsibility.

DEVELOP APPROACHES

Plan approaches that are uniquely related to the resident's strengths, weaknesses, problems, and needs. During the care plan meeting, discussion among members focuses experience and expertise towards development of individualized approaches or helping strategies for each resident. Use approaches as a way to take into account the idiosyncrasies of the resident and to incorporate the personal touch, which individualizes care for every resident.

Approaches must reflect the uniqueness of the resident, facility, and staff. For example, the care plan team must take into account the special helping talents of an activity aide as they develop

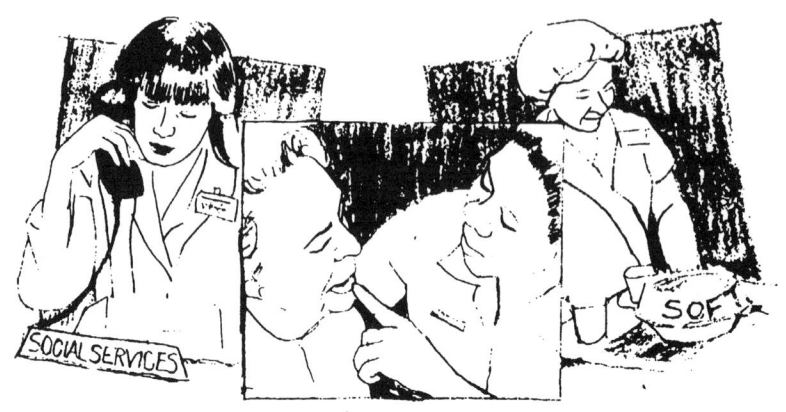

FIGURE 6.1 Goal achievement relies on interdisciplinary approaches.

approaches to a resident's activity goal. Let the approaches do the best job for the resident by making the best use of facility, staff, and resident resources. (See Figure 6.1.)

LIST THE APPROACHES

Write the developed approaches on the care plan under a designated heading called "approaches." Group the approaches with each respective problem, need, and goal.

ASSIGN RESPONSIBILITY

Several approaches are often written in support of a single goal with responsibility assigned to staff members or departments. For example, the care plan team identifies a resident problem area as "weight loss, eating difficulties."

Problem: weight loss, eating difficulties.
Approaches:
1. Social Services—Contact family or state agency for funding to buy dentures.
2. Nursing—CNA assigned to resident will assist resident at meal time by cutting food and helping resident to eat by using hand-over-hand guidance for each meal.
3. Dietary—Serve snacks three times per day consisting of either cheese and crackers, cookies, or small sandwiches.

Each responsible department utilizes its assigned approach when working with a resident towards attainment of the goal.

Chapter 7

IMPLEMENTATION

Implementation is delivering the specific care, as presented by the care plan, to the resident. During implementation, the care plan is transformed from a mere document to an active and focused treatment. A consistent day after day philosophy helps to ensure delivery of care as indicated by the care plan.

These four steps of implementation lend vitality to the delivery of care as indicated by the care plan:

1. Communicate the care plan to all staff.
2. Provide innovative support.
3. Monitor the delivery.
4. Fine tune the care plan or its delivery.

COMMUNICATE THE CARE PLAN TO ALL STAFF

Communication is essential to build knowledge of the care plan among the caregivers. The caregivers must know the resident's care plan before they can offer care which reflects that plan. Responsibility for the implementation of care as indicated by the care plan must reach from the care plan team to the direct providers of care who are, in most cases, the nurse's aides.

Communication of the care plan can take written or verbal form. In homes which have exemplary care plans, a written document, such as a care card or care checklist sheet, is placed in the hands of the responsible care delivery person(s). A resident's goals and approaches are listed on the care card or care checklist sheet. This written document is passed from shift to shift, from aide to aide, from hand to hand. The content of the care plan reaches the people who deliver the care through the use of written forms.

Communication forms used by different facilities vary but they share common characteristics. For example, many communication forms incorporate a section for direct care providers to document progress toward each care plan goal; however, all communication forms tell direct care providers the approaches and goals for a resident. They serve to improve the flow of information from the care plan team to the direct care providers.

Two examples of communication forms are "Care Cards" and a "Goal Checksheet."

Care Cards

Care cards are used to list the goals and approaches indicated in the care plan. Care cards are carried by the aides in their pockets for easy reference. Cards are passed between shifts along with any important information regarding the resident's performance in these goal areas. These cards provide an important communication option to the care plan team and can be effective with a minimum of effort.

Management staff must show commitment to the use of care cards by instructing direct caregivers about a resident's goals and approach. Just because the cards are in the caregiver's pocket does not mean that they are read or referenced as needed. A way of assuring staff knowledge and action towards resident goals is to require staff documentation. Require staff to document the care that was provided which reflects the care plan. With expectations clearly shown, and support provided, the caregivers will expend great efforts to use care cards and implement the care plan.

- Revise and update care cards at the care plan meeting.
- Replace all cards as needed to prevent the circulation of unreadable cards. Care cards that are carried by the caregivers will rapidly deteriorate unless they are wrapped in plastic or

otherwise protected. Baths, cleaning compounds, food, and day-to-day handling eventually make unprotected cards unreadable.
- Transfer care cards between shifts according to work assignment. The cards available to a caregiver will correspond to his/her workload or assignment.

An example of a care card can be found in Appendix I.

Goal Checksheet

On a goal checksheet, goals and approaches are listed in one column on a page, with space provided to mark which approaches were carried out on a daily basis. These sheets are stored in the residents' charts or in notebooks grouped by hallway, floor, or assignment. Caregivers document daily on the sheets by marking the approaches they carried out with each resident and by noting the progress the resident has made toward attaining each goal. Employees will quickly learn the approaches and goals if they are required to mark or document care delivery actions. As with the care card and any other tool, management effort is necessary to make them effective.

- The goal checksheet is more sophisticated than the care card and requires more instruction and administrative support for effective use. In-services must be provided to instruct staff about using this form. Instructions for marking the frequency on the correct day, determining what constitutes resident behavior towards a goal, and when to mark the behavior are possible in-service topics.
- Revise goal checksheets at the care plan meeting. When the care plan is developed, goals and approaches are recorded on a clean checksheet.
- Store the goal checksheets on the unit. A care delivery worker must be able to quickly access the goal checksheets. Divide the books by floor, wing, or work assignment.
- Time must be allocated for staff to document resident actions towards goals. If time is specifically set aside for the checksheets, the documentation will be more consistent and accurate.

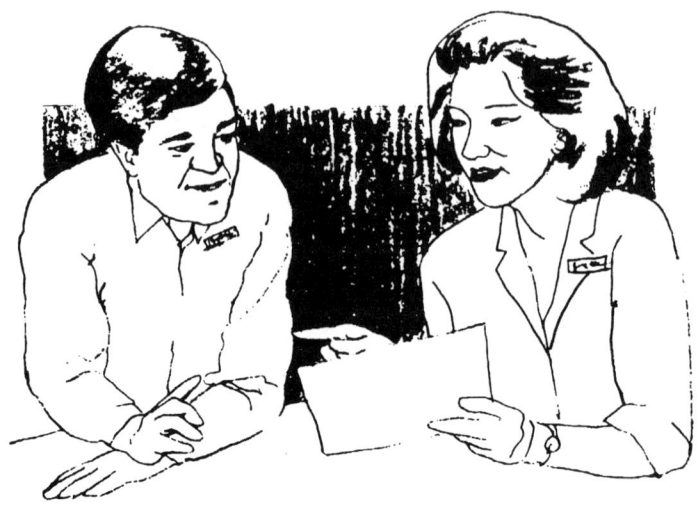

FIGURE 7.1 Verbal communication is important to ensure proper care.

An example of a Goal Checksheet can be found in Appendix J.

Verbal communication of the care plan is the simplest method to ensure that direct providers of care are knowledgeable about the care plan. In the verbal form, a supervisor tells a direct care provider about the resident's care plan. (See Figure 7.1.) Supportive reminders may be offered to ensure that the direct provider remembers the approaches and goals. All staff who have contact with the resident must be told about the care plan.

In verbally communicating the care plan, the following should be considered:

- It may be most effective to discuss care plan goals with the aide while the aide is engaged in the goal oriented activity with the resident. For example, if an aide is assisting a resident in eating, it is effective to inform the aide that the resident's goal is to eat at least 75% of her food. Also, inform the aide of approaches to help the resident eat as detailed in the care plan. The aide will now know that the resident's goal is to eat 75% of her food, and the aide will know how to help the resident achieve the goal.

Implementation 41

- Continually offer reminders about care plan goals and approaches to staff. Offer suggestions with sensitivity to the staff member's pride, self-esteem, and concept of their own competence. Inform staff of revisions in the resident's care plan.

PROVIDE INNOVATIVE SUPPORT

Making a commitment to deliver the care plan services requires administrative and management support. Support can be as easy to provide as giving compliments to staff who conscientiously provide goal-directed care. Noticing and remarking on improvements in resident abilities is an incentive to staff members to continue to expend effort in assisting residents.

Administrative or management innovations indicate a commitment to deliver the care plan services. Some examples of management support, by no means exhaustive, include permanently assigning aides to residents, initiating aide documentation, and overlapping shifts. Each of these management innovations supports consistent delivery of the care plan.

Permanent Assignment

This is a program which ensures that aides are familiar with their assigned residents. Aides are assigned to work with the same group of residents on a continual basis. A stable work assignment means that the aide is more familiar with and committed to the resident's care plan.

Aide Documentation

Activity, rehabilitative, and nurse's aides record daily care. This assures that care specific to the care plan is being given, and provides a record to justify an alteration of the care approaches or goals if necessary.

Overlapping Shifts

Schedule an overlap between shifts so that certain tasks are finished more quickly (many jobs go quicker with two workers, such as making beds or giving bed baths to skilled care residents). The staff time saved by overlapping shifts can be used to implement programs such as decubitus care, passive range of motion, or activities of daily living.

MONITOR THE DELIVERY

The implementation process is incomplete without a monitoring procedure. Monitoring assures quality and creates a communication feedback loop for problems that might otherwise go undetected. Monitoring assures the effective implementation of the care plan by identifying difficulties that can then be solved. Information for monitoring purposes may be gathered from residents, written documentation, observations, or from staff.

FINE-TUNE THE CARE PLAN OR ITS DELIVERY

If information sources show that a resident is not meeting a goal, then a follow-up to assess alternative goals and approaches is necessary. A reassessment process should be made and, if necessary, alterations in the care plan should be discussed during an interdisciplinary care plan meeting. Incorporate these changes into a modified care plan.

Chapter 8

DOCUMENTATION

Documentation is the written description of care and services that have been provided to a resident according to the care plan. Documentation:

- Describes a condition
- States what services have been provided
- Describes a resident's accomplishments
- Provides a baseline against which to monitor progress
- Is a communication instrument to be used among staff and between shifts and departments.

Many homes provide excellent care to their residents, but few accurately and comprehensively describe the care residents receive. Exemplary homes prove their caring actions through descriptive writing, which then becomes a valuable source in providing current care and in planning future care. Care planners use documentation to evaluate and show evidence of progress toward care plan goals. The steps of care plan documentation are:

1. Require all staff to document.
2. Document using a consistent format.
3. Document daily.
4. Write periodic summaries.
5. Make documentation accessible to staff.

REQUIRE ALL STAFF TO DOCUMENT

Direct care providers are best equipped to report on care delivery and resident's responses to care delivery because they personally perform the care delivery tasks. For example, it is the nurse's aide who knows from one day to the next whether or not the resident is becoming better able to walk a certain distance or is able to wash his or her own legs. It is the aide's responsibility to record such data on a daily basis. Each department has separate documentation forms for the resident.

DOCUMENT USING A CONSISTENT FORMAT

Effective documentation does two things within a prescribed format: it describes the action of the caregiver, and it describes the reaction of the resident. Using a certain format and following guidelines makes documentation more effective. Documentation guidelines include:

- Date of documentation
- Title of documentation note in the margin, e.g., social service progress note, nursing monthly summary, nursing incident report
- Problem/need relevant to the note
- Action and approach of the caregiver
- Resident reactions to the care and approach
- Results of the care offered
- Recommendations about more effective approaches and precautions to remember concerning the resident
- Signature or initials and title of writer.

Documentation example:

Activities Monthly Summary 7/29/92
Mr. X has a problem of sleeping in chairs and slipping to the floor. He was escorted from the reception area three times during the first week of this month due to sleeping. He complains to the nurse's aide that he

is not tired when they escort him to his room, but quickly falls asleep after lying down in bed. To limit these chair sleeping incidents to no more than once per week, Mr. X has been successfully engaged three times a week in morning coffee chats with other residents and in afternoon group activities. Since the approach was initiated on 7/22, Mr. X has only had one sleeping incident.

Signed,
Name, Title

Behavioral terms represent the only concrete means to record what is happening to the resident. It is only through behaviors that indications of changes in feelings or condition may be measured. For example, a social worker cannot state that a resident is less depressed; however, he or she may note indications of reduced depression by documenting that the resident cried only two times during a certain period, as compared with a similar period when the resident cried five times.

DOCUMENT DAILY

The day-to-day record is critical as a basis to evaluate achievement of goals. Daily recording legitimizes claims of progress toward care plan goals, which are otherwise difficult to remember over a long period of time. To assure accurate daily documentation, staff must record events as they occur or before the end of the shift.

WRITE PERIODIC SUMMARIES

Periodic summaries record the patterns of resident accomplishments and responses to the care plan. Summaries give an overall picture of how the resident has progressed toward goals and what approaches have proven to be effective. These summaries, written by department supervisors, become a planning tool for use by the care plan team while evaluating old goals and developing new goals. Sources of information for these summaries include: daily notes, previous summary notes, incident reports, bath sheets, nursing reports, dietary intake charts, etc.

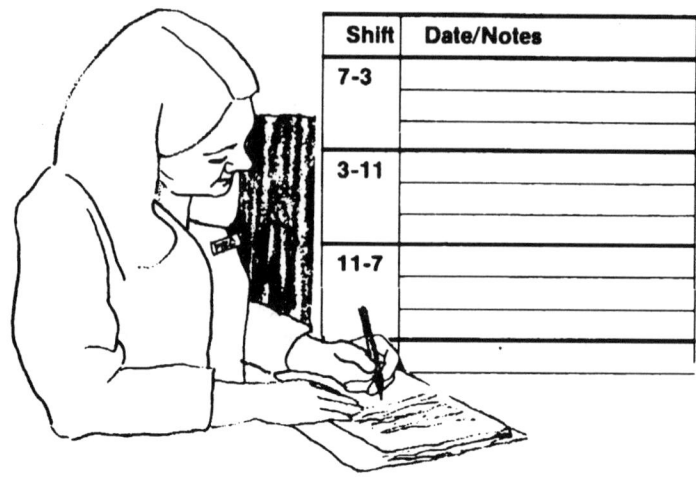

FIGURE 8.1 Documentation is an important, ongoing process.

MAKE DOCUMENTATION ACCESSIBLE TO STAFF

For ease of daily recording and referral, locate documentation forms at the nurse's station in charts or data books so that all staff can access the forms without leaving their resident work assignment. Organize the forms by resident, floor, unit, or assignment.

Chapter **9**

EVALUATION

Evaluation is the last step of the care planning process. During this formal review process, each goal listed on the care plan is examined to determine whether the resident has achieved it or not. The responsible department reviews the resident's chart and makes a decision about goal achievement. In addition, consultation occurs with the resident, family members, other staff, and any other person who may have information about the resident's goal achievement.

Follow this formal review process to evaluate goals:

1. Gather data about goal performance.
2. Establish goal achievement status.
3. Document the goal achievement status.
4. Discuss the reasons for the goal status.

GATHER DATA ABOUT GOAL PERFORMANCE

The care plan team member needs to systematically gather information about a resident's performance on the care plan goals shortly before the scheduled revision. The data that are to be examined include:

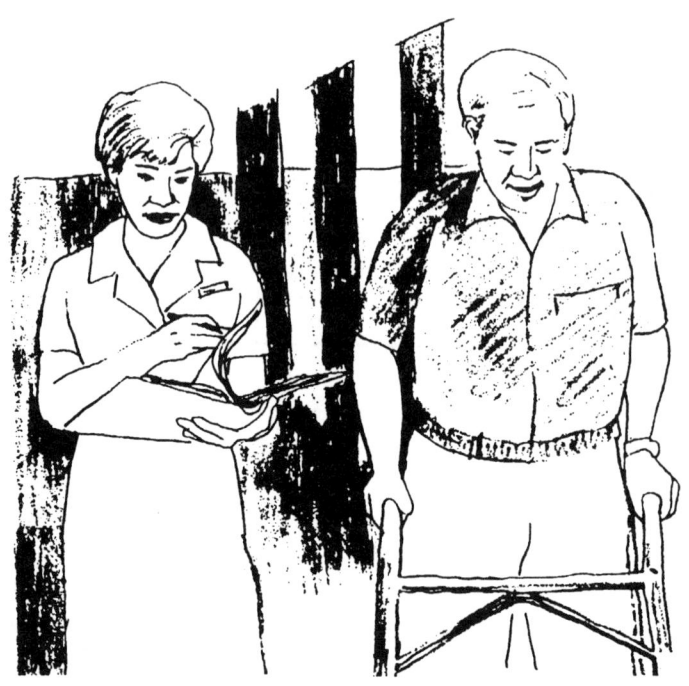

FIGURE 9.1 Direct observation of goal related activity.

- Objective statements such as lab results, progress notes, nursing reports, etc.
- Subjective expressions from the resident, family, or staff (e.g., "Mother seems so much happier since...")
- Direct observation of the resident engaged in goal related activity or task. (See Figure 9.1.)

ESTABLISH GOAL ACHIEVEMENT STATUS

Goal achievement status is established by analyzing the objective and subjective data collected. One way to evaluate how residents are meeting their goals is to turn the goal into a question. If the goal is that the resident will eat independently, then the question becomes, "Is the resident eating independently?"

Scan the information for indications of sustained performance or maintenance of the desired goal levels over the time frame period.

DOCUMENT THE GOAL ACHIEVEMENT STATUS

Use a standard notation method to document goal achievement or nonachievement as determined by the evaluation process. Record the goal status on the care plan. A clear notation system will reveal the goal status at a single glance.

DISCUSS REASONS FOR THE GOAL STATUS

During the care plan meeting, discuss the effectiveness of the approaches and the appropriateness of the goals given the resident's strengths, weaknesses, and the facility's resources. If an acceptable level of progress has not been reached at the time of review, then the resident and care plan team must evaluate what is blocking the progress. Questions to ask may include:

- Is the resident invested in this goal?
- Do team members carry out the approaches in a consistent manner?
- Are approaches effective?
- Is the goal specific, realistic, and measurable?

Chapter 10

CONCLUSION

Good care planning is essential for providing quality care to residents in long-term care facilities. This manual describes the care planning process and provides guidelines that long-term care facilities can use in providing care to their residents. Facilities are encouraged to consider implementing the suggestions in this manual as they create optimal care planning processes that serve their residents' needs.

A care planning process checklist is provided after this statement for staff convenience. The process checklist is to be used as a guide for the creation of a customized care planning process for individual facilities:

ASSESSMENT

- Learn about resident before admission.
- Inform each department of a new resident.
- Assign responsibility for the assessment.
- Collect information.
- Identify problems, needs, and strengths.
- Continue ongoing assessment.
- Perform reassessment periodically.

CARE PLAN MEETING

- Create a productive setting.
- Develop a meeting schedule.
- Select an interdisciplinary team.
- Involve residents and family members.
- Designate a care plan coordinator.
- Delegate duties among team members.
- Evaluate previous goals.
- Record information on the care plan form.
- Discuss the resident's problems, needs, and strengths.

GOALS

- Develop goals that measure progress towards solving a resident's problems and fulfilling the resident's needs.
- Keep goals in mind when delivering care.
- State goals in realistic, behavioral, and measurable terms.

APPROACHES

- Develop approaches.
- List the approaches on the care plan.
- Assign responsibility to a staff person or department.
- Document resident responses to approaches.

IMPLEMENTATION

- Communicate the care plan to all staff.
- Provide supportive resources to implement the care plan.
- Monitor the care plan delivery.
- Fine-tune the care plan or its delivery as necessary.

DOCUMENTATION

- Require all staff to document their actions and resident's responses.
- Document using a consistent format.
- Document daily.
- Write periodic summaries.
- Make documentation accessible to staff.

EVALUATION

- Gather data about resident's performance.
- Establish goal achievement status.
- Document goal achievement status.
- Discuss reasons for status.

PART II

QUALITY ASSURANCE

INTRODUCTION

Health care in nursing homes has traditionally followed the "medical model." Staffed with medical personnel in hospital-like buildings, facilities have tended to focus primarily on the medical needs of "patients." This section proposes that facilities take a more holistic approach to resident care by developing and implementing quality assurance programs. This means that in addition to medical needs, the social, cognitive, and spiritual needs of the residents are also addressed.

An effective quality assurance program can help nursing home personnel identify problems in meeting the needs of residents and provide an organized approach to resolving those problems. The outcome is an improved quality of life for the residents and, because quality of life issues have a direct effect on the families of residents, an effective quality assurance program also benefits families who can take comfort in knowing that the facility is delivering the best possible care to their loved ones.

The benefits of a successful quality assurance program are not limited to nursing home residents and their families. Working conditions for staff are enhanced by providing them with clearly defined expectations for job performance, by encouraging them to participate in decisions that affect their jobs, and by creating an atmosphere of cooperation in accordance with the home's philosophy of care.

Part II has been designed to provide you, the nursing home employee, with information about quality assurance in nursing homes. A working definition of quality assurance will be developed, two types of quality assurance programs will be discussed, the benefits of a good quality assurance program will be addressed, and variables in the makeup of a facility that determine the selection of an appropriate quality assurance program will be suggested. As you read, consider quality assurance in your facility, and how your job contributes to quality assurance.

Chapter 11

WHAT IS QUALITY ASSURANCE?

Quality assurance in nursing homes is the set of procedures a facility uses to promote excellence in the provision of care.

Quality refers to the specific performance standards or goals a facility sets as levels of achievement to be maintained.

Assurance refers to the process of guaranteeing that quality is achieved and maintained. Assurance procedures consist of these four steps:

1. *Identifying* needs and formulating goals for meeting needs and then *identifying* reasons for the difference between actual performance and desired quality performance
2. *Planning* what needs to be done to bring performance up to quality standards
3. *Implementing* changes that help bring performance up to quality levels
4. *Evaluating* the extent to which the desired quality of performance is achieved.

Quality assurance procedures are ongoing and dynamic. This means that quality assurance is not a one-time or stop-and-start effort. It is a cyclical process (see Figure 11.1) that must be maintained to achieve the desired excellence in service.

Quality assurance in nursing homes takes the form of systematic programs designed to *identify* problems in care delivery, formulate *plans* to correct the problems, *implement* the plans, and *evalu-*

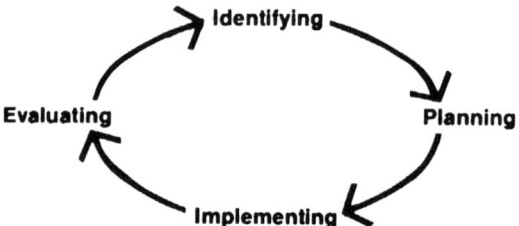

FIGURE 11.1 The quality assurance cycle.

ate the outcome to determine if the plans were effective in eliminating the problems. An effective quality assurance program maintains the cyclical process described above.

To give the definition of quality assurance utility, the remainder of this manual is devoted to examining the impact of quality assurance by considering and answering the following questions:

- Does quality assurance mean quality care of residents?
- How does quality assurance affect administrators, supervisors, and staff?
- How does quality assurance create a positive community image of the nursing home?
- How does quality assurance benefit the families of residents?
- How can quality assurance improve the nursing home's physical environment?
- Is quality assurance cost effective?
- Is quality assurance attainable?

Chapter 12

DOES QUALITY ASSURANCE MEAN QUALITY CARE?

THE QUALITY OF LIFE MISSION

The first step in developing a successful quality assurance program is to identify the specific standards the facility desires to achieve. Research on organizational development and success has found a strong relationship between an organization's sense of purpose or mission and the quality of the organizational culture and the service it delivers. When goals are clearly interwoven and reinforced within all aspects of an organizational climate, employees naturally begin to internalize the value system of the mission and to function more smoothly as an integrated unit.

Mission goals of nursing homes are usually developed by the owner, administrator, and directors of the various departments. However, innovative facilities may want to ask all staff, volunteers, residents, and families to participate in offering their suggestions for mission goals. This way, a diversity of valuable ideas is obtained, and many persons are uplifted as their self-worth is enhanced through the process.

A careful and thorough assessment of the characteristics, expectations, and needs of the residents can help the facility develop a mission statement of quality of life standards that staff and residents can aim for and achieve. For example, nursing home residents typically have a wide range of medical, physical, psychological, emotional, cognitive, and spiritual disabilities and needs. Their independence and social and environmental activities are limited as well. They are characteristically single, have no children living close by, and are poorer than the population in general. Taking the example further, from this description of resident characteristics, disabilities, and needs combined with a basic ethical sense of human needs, several general quality of life standards for residents can be generated. It is important that residents:

- Feel a sense of well-being, self-worth, and self-esteem
- Feel a sense of satisfaction with their care
- Enjoy a medically sound and safe physical environment
- Have the opportunity to have close and meaningful relationships with others
- Are able to achieve desired goals and exercise choice
- Enjoy a sense of privacy, dignity, and reasonable control over life decisions.

This list, of course, is only partial. Many holistic quality of life standards for residents will be generated by each facility. Each facility will also reflect its own unique sense of mission and philosophy of quality of life for its residents.

TRANSLATING THE QUALITY OF LIFE MISSION

A facility that delivers excellent service to its residents is one that is able to *enthusiastically translate its sense of quality of life mission to its entire staff*. (See Figure 12.1.) Ideals or goals of quality of life for residents are not static or contained merely within the pages of a notebook. Rather, they are *enthusiastically* conveyed to the staff and residents by the administrator and department heads. They are conveyed:

- In a positive, uplifting manner
- On a day-by-day, ongoing basis
- In a dynamic way that is continually open to change, input, and growth

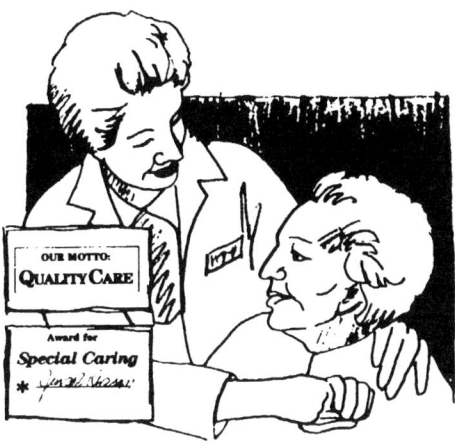

FIGURE 12.1 Nursing home mission clearly stated will be carried out by staff.

- In a trusting sense that staff will carry out their goals in a responsible way.

The quality of life goals or mission statement of a facility can be kept alive and fostered through creative ways of expressing them on an ongoing basis. Some ideas that have proven successful include enlivening the social climate of the facility by expressing the mission goals in:

- Memos to department heads concerning procedures
  – Describe how new procedures support the goals of the facility.
  – Show how deleted procedures no longer support the goals.
- Staff meetings
  – The general foundation for discussions can be the home's mission goals.
  – Show how problems detract from facility goals and ask for solutions that support them.
- Ways of showing appreciation
  – Send flowers or a plant to a department that is doing an outstanding job. Include a note describing how the work promotes the mission of the nursing home.

-When giving individual employees "pats on the back." tell them how their good work supports the home's mission.
- A general statement on facility stationery that summarizes the home's mission goals
- Goals engraved on a plaque hung in the reception area
- Statements of the mission goals given to all job applicants and to new personnel during orientation
  -Give job applicants a printed copy expressing goals.
  -Verbally explain the goals during the first day of orientation.

In the nursing home, quality assurance means delivering quality care and service to the residents. Staff who understand, agree with, and appreciate the overall mission of their facility will be better able to work together cooperatively to provide the best possible care and service to the residents.

Chapter **13**

HOW DOES QUALITY ASSURANCE AFFECT MANAGEMENT AND STAFF?

In many long-term care facilities, it is the administrator in conjunction with department supervisors who sets levels of expectations for all the different jobs that must be done if quality care is to be delivered to the residents. Administrators and supervisors are necessarily influenced by external regulatory agencies to set standards that are in harmony with laws that govern licensure and certification. Standards of care that go above and beyond those laws may be set by managers either in or outside the facility. In facilities where job expectations are set by someone outside the facility, such as board members or corporate executives, it is still the responsibility of the administrator and the supervisors to ensure that those expectations are being met.

Meeting expectations in care delivery means that problems, or potential problems, must be quickly and accurately identified and resolved. Problem identification, assessment, and resolution are largely managerial tasks; however, all staff can participate in the problem solving process. A successful quality assurance program encourages staff to speak up with new ideas and to become involved in solving problems that affect their own jobs as well as other departments in the facility. Administrators and supervisors benefit from the fresh insight and staff are given a sense of power and control over their jobs.

The grand objective of a quality assurance program is to eliminate problems in resident care. It is unrealistic to expect that *all* possible problems that can occur in a nursing home can be eliminated. However, a sound quality assurance program can significantly reduce the number and severity of the problems that inevitably arise so that excellence in care, as defined by the facility, is achieved and maintained.

Administrators and supervisors can help staff to do their best possible work by following these four guidelines:

1. Make job expectations clear to staff.
   - During orientation give each new employee a written and clearly defined job description that includes performance standards acceptable to the facility. (See Appendix L for a sample job description.)
   - Make clear to each employee the consequences of not meeting job performance standards.
   - Consequences should include, but not be limited to, disciplinary or termination issues.
   - Explain to each employee how his or her job contributes to quality care of the residents and how failure to meet facility standards not only results in poor quality care, but can also jeopardize the employee's well-being.
   - Give all employees access to copies of the various job descriptions throughout the facility with quality performance criteria.
2. Schedule regular meetings between staff and management.
   - Encourage employee input regarding problems and solutions or innovative ideas in care. Use their various perspectives and talents to gain fresh insight into care delivery.
   - Invite employees to role play problems and solutions as a fun way of creating and developing new ideas. (See Appendix M for an example.)
   - Give verbal "trivia" quizzes on facility policies, standards, and procedures. Give a prize to the employee who answers the most questions correctly.
   - Record and post minutes from the meetings for all employees to read. (See Appendix N for an example.)
3. Give employees incentives for contributing to quality assurance.
   - Recognize good work with "pats on the back" and plenty of verbal "thank yous."

- Put a suggestion box in the employees' lounge or other places where employees eat or take breaks and reward employees whose suggestions are implemented. (See Appendix O for examples of suggestions contributed by employees.) Suggested rewards include:
  –Small monetary rewards
  –Time off from work with pay
  –Recognition by putting employee's picture and suggestion on a bulletin board in a prominent place in the facility.
- Celebrate successful evaluations by supervisors with parties or gifts such as new plants or flowers for the departments.

4. Schedule regular employee evaluations.
   - Schedule evaluations in addition to the evaluations done for the purpose of increasing wages to give employees feedback on how well they are performing their jobs. (See Appendix P for sample job evaluation.)
   - Evaluations should emphasize strong as well as weak points in job performance.
   - Leave space on the evaluation form for employees to respond.
   - Evaluations can be written by a team of supervisors so that no one supervisor must carry the responsibility if negative comments must be made.
   - If evaluations are discussed between the administrator or the DON and the employee, give the written evaluation to the employee a day before the conference so that he or she will have time to think about and react to the evaluation.
   - Have an "employee of the month" election. Employees can vote using ballots that include space for why the employee is being nominated. Put winners' names on a bulletin board in a prominent place in the facility along with a list of the qualities from the ballots that make him or her an outstanding employee.

Employees can significantly contribute to quality assurance in a facility if they are allowed to become an important and integral part of the facility's quality assurance program (see Figure 13.1). Employees who have a clear understanding of what needs to be done and how to do it will be less at risk for making mistakes

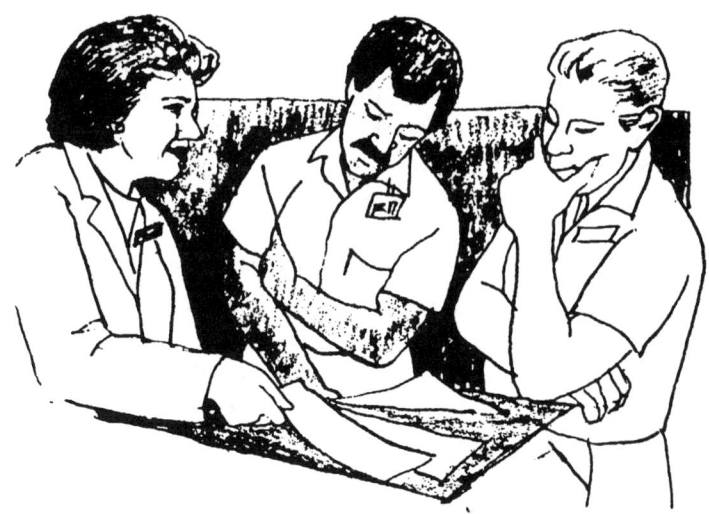

FIGURE 13.1 Quality assurance is a team effort.

because of ignorance concerning job standards and procedures. Supervisors and administrators will benefit because they will need to spend less time disciplining employees who have created problems and, with the additional input of the employees, less time trying to identify and solve problems. Also, when employees are allowed to contribute to decisions affecting their jobs, either verbally in meetings or by seeing their written suggestions implemented, the resulting sense of pride and ownership in the facility will promote an atmosphere of teamwork and rapport among the employees, making the facility a happier place to be for everyone.

Employees who feel they are members of a team sharing the responsibilities of quality care delivery to the residents will naturally work together more cooperatively than employees who feel isolated in their jobs. A sense of teamwork and community within the facility can be fostered by administrators and supervisors who present themselves as members of the team *by their actions.* Managers who are perceived as "doers" by staff, i.e. as participating members of a team with a common objective, will help staff to achieve high quality job performance because:

- Staff are more comfortable interacting with managers with whom they have daily contact than with managers they see only occasionally.

- Staff feel that managers understand their jobs and can appreciate the difficulty and stress that accompanies their work.
- Staff are more inspired to work when they see their managers working.
- Staff can get to know managers on a more personal basis, making them more approachable when problems need to be discussed.

Encouraging staff to interact with managers can help involve staff in decision making and problem solving procedures. The following ideas may help to integrate management and staff into a comfortable, cooperative, and mutually respectful working relationship:

- Managers and staff can take coffee or lunch breaks together.
- Managers can keep an "open door policy," which means that they are always available to staff.
- Managers and staff can be encouraged to greet each other by name in and outside of the facility.
- Management and staff can have at least one task they do together, such as feeding residents or making beds.

These ideas can help to create an atmosphere of teamwork in the nursing home. Sharing activities and responsibilities with their managers can help to increase staff morale. Staff and residents alike will benefit from the happier and more home-like environment.

Chapter **14**

HOW DOES QUALITY ASSURANCE CREATE A POSITIVE COMMUNITY IMAGE?

By moving away from the medical model of nursing homes to a holistic care plan model, the nursing home becomes more of a home to the people who live there and less like an institution in which they are housed. Because the residents of the facility are also citizens of the community in which it is located, quality of life issues analyzed from the perspectives of the residents must not fail to consider the relationship between the nursing home and the community.

How the facility is perceived by the community can have a bearing on the residents' feelings of well-being, self-worth, and self-esteem. At some point before moving into the facility each resident was most likely living independently in a community setting, freely interacting with the other members of that community. While it may not be realistic to expect that residents are able to remain as active in the community as they once were, it is possible to create and promote feelings of community membership by developing a positive and active relationship between the community and the facility. (See Figure 14.1.) This can help to alleviate the feelings of abandonment and isolation that residents report experiencing when they move from their own familiar homes to the new and often frightening facility environment. Developing an active relationship between the facility and the community means more than simply transporting the residents from the facility into the com-

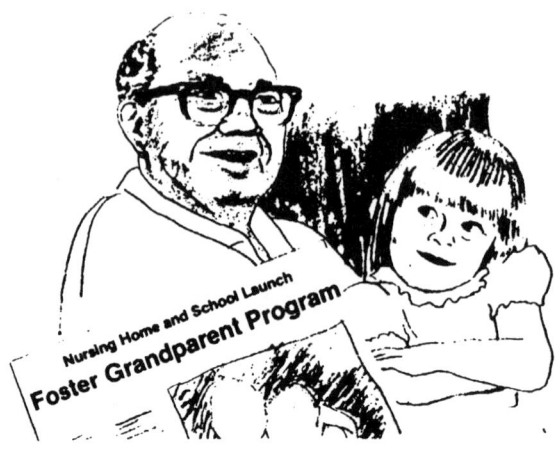

FIGURE 14.1 Nursing home is an integral part of the community.

munity. While this is indeed crucial to establishing good facility-community relations, it is also important that members of the community interact with the residents in the facility.

To encourage citizens of the community to visit, the facility should present itself not as an isolated entity but as a vital and dynamic member of the larger community system. To achieve this image the facility must inform and educate the community about the residents who live there, its philosophy of care, and the interesting programs that are being developed or implemented. In addition, the needs of the facility and how community people can contribute to and benefit from visiting the facility, either casually or as participants in a formal volunteer program, must be communicated. The following are suggestions for educating and informing the community about the nursing home:

- Link up the facility with the community social service network. Workers may be interested or know clients who are interested in volunteering services or donating material goods to the facility. Also, agencies may be willing to include information about the facility in their newsletters and bulletins.
- Look for someone in the facility who could give talks on aging, long-term care, or other topics related to the facility.

- Publish articles in the local newspapers about the facility and what is happening there. (See Appendix Q for topic ideas.)
- Advertise volunteer opportunities on grocery store bulletin boards or on flyers posted in churches or with other prominent community organizations.
- Develop an educational program with schools so that students can learn about the aging process by interacting with the residents in the facility, by telephone, through letters, or by visiting.
- Children can make valuable contributions to the facility's volunteer program and add a special dimension to the lives of the residents. Encourage children to volunteer time and service to the home by sending someone from the facility to the schools to describe to the children what jobs they can do to help the residents and staff. Also, encourage the children to create their own ideas for volunteer service.
- Sponsor a local Retired Seniors Volunteer Program (RSVP) so that volunteers work out of the facility, or have the facility serve as a volunteer station where RSVP members can volunteer.

There are many other ways a facility can create community interest; these are only a few suggestions. By taking a public relations approach, the facility can actively and successfully recruit volunteers, educate the public about the aging process, promote a positive attitude toward the nursing home, and, most importantly, enhance the lives of the residents who have made the facility their home.

Chapter 15

HOW DOES QUALITY ASSURANCE BENEFIT FAMILIES?

What responsibilities does a nursing home have to the families of residents? Although the primary commitment of care is to the resident, facilities that adopt the holistic care plan model suggested in this manual will strive to create a facility environment in which families can feel comfortable expressing concern and loving support for their family members.

Families typically make the decision to institutionalize their relatives only after exhausting all other resources. Because families tend to have strong desires to maintain their relatives at home, the institutionalization process is often experienced as a crisis. Families are forced to confront the harsh realities of a loved one's illness, the pain of a separation that restructures the family, and the inevitable mortality of their relative and themselves. At the height of this crisis the family admits their relative to a nursing home for care that they cannot give at home.

Nursing home staff first encounter the new resident's family during this pivotal point in the family's life. At this critical time the needs of the family must be recognized and met so that their relative's transition into the home is made as easily and as smoothly as possible for everyone involved in the process. Staff can help the resident's family by providing them with:

- Kind and gentle emotional support
  - Recognize that the family is experiencing a crisis.
  - Find out what expectations the family has of the facility and reassure them that reasonable expectations will be met.
  - Remain aware that families often experience conflicting feelings about placing their relatives in nursing homes and their behavior may reflect the conflict.
- Respect for the care they have given their relative so far and the opportunity to remain involved in caring
  - Encourage families to visit the facility.
  - Tell them about activities they can participate in such as helping to feed residents or other volunteer opportunities.
  - Invite them to participate in the care planning process.
  - Put their names on mailing lists for any newsletters or bulletins put out by the nursing home.

Families can be valuable contributors to the well-being of residents and the nursing home in general (see Figure 15.1). On the other hand, if proper care and attention are not given to families, they can become effective saboteurs of staff and resident morale. For example, management problems arise when there is conflict between residents and fam-

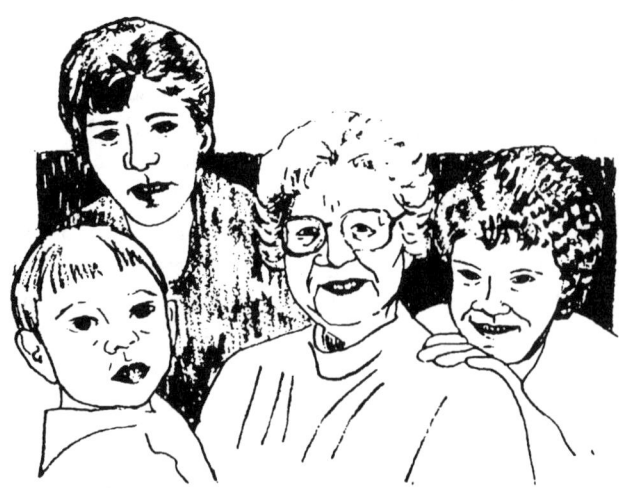

FIGURE 15.1 Families are valuable contributors to the well-being of residents.

ily members, and intervening staff may often wind up as convenient scapegoats. Family members may also experience considerable denial or guilt which can result in emotional over-reactions, rejections, and distortions of the resident's behavior, illness, and/or reduced prospects for their relative's recovery.

Family members can have unrealistic expectations of both resident and staff behavior that will lead to further conflict. If families do not understand the reasons for staff actions, or feel put off and without input, the resulting poor family–staff interaction will have unfortunate consequences for everyone, especially the residents.

Nursing homes that strive for excellence in holistic care can create quality assurance programs in the area of family care. The optimum quality assurance program for enhancing family crisis resolution and family/staff/resident integration is one that *actively recruits and serves the family as a client of the nursing home*. Policies that promote family well-being are also likely to have positive effects on residents and staff members alike.

Implementation of a quality assurance program that actively involves the families of residents as clients need not be viewed as a costly endeavor. Most aspects of a family quality assurance program are not costly, can actually increase staff efficiency, improve the community image, and promote resident/family satisfaction.

The first step in setting up a family quality assurance program is to carefully and thoroughly *identify the characteristics and needs of the families*. Characteristics and needs can be surveyed through:

- Observation
- Interviews with residents and their families
- Surveys or questionnaires
- Relevant books and articles

The second step is to *plan* policies and specific programs and procedures to meet family needs. Some examples of programs and procedures that actively involve families in resident care are:

- Family group counseling sessions which optimally include all members of the newly admitted resident's family. These sessions are usually conducted by trained social workers and are designed to allow families to express their feelings regarding the placement of their relative in the nursing home.

The sessions help both the resident and the family adjust more easily to the new situation and decrease conflict and guilt that can make the separation more problematic.
- Inclusion of the family in a comprehensive psychiatric assessment of the newly admitted resident. Inclusion of the family is essential for a complete understanding of the resident. This collaboration values family input and involves the family in important considerations of resident care. Collaboration can also help families to come to terms with unresolved issues and can lead to greater adaptation and emotional openness within the entire family.
- Community support groups for families engaged in decision making about the care of the frail elderly. Lead by nurses or social workers, these groups help families make difficult decisions, deal with anxiety and negative emotions, and cope effectively with their concerns. These groups can be purely supportive and/or educational and social, and can help families alleviate some of their feelings of isolation, guilt, grief, frustration, confusion, and helplessness. They can also train families in care skills, quality visitation skills, and in understanding the developmental issues of the aging process.
- Periodic written communication to families concerning the progress of their relatives to reduce anxiety, especially for families who are unable to visit the facility on a regular basis. Personalized letters sent out two or three times a year keep families informed about and help them to feel involved in the lives of their relatives. (See Appendix R for an example of a letter to a family.)

Research indicates that most families need and welcome programs and classes that can increase their communication and visiting skills as well as their understanding of the aging process. Examples of specific educational program topics include:

- Organic brain disease
- Mood disturbances
- Mental and physical deterioration
- The process of aging and institutionalization
- Death and dying
- Alzheimer's disease

- Medication
- Activities and exercise

Scheduled activities for families are an important aspect of dynamic family involvement. Some suggestions for family activities are:

- Monthly coffee houses for family and staff
- Resident/staff/family parties on holidays
- Community outings for residents and families
- A committee of family members to help design facility policies
- Surveys and questionnaires to solicit family suggestions and/ or complaints concerning the nursing home.

The particular components of a family quality assurance program will, of course, differ according to the particular strengths and needs of each facility. Once those strengths and needs are *identified*, activities and programs can be designed and *implemented*. The final step in creating a family quality assurance program is *evaluating* the effectiveness of the activities and programs. Evaluative measures that may indicate the success of a program include:

- Decrease of staff/family/resident conflicts
- Increase in family visits
- Decrease in family complaints
- Decrease in unrealistic expectations of families
- Increase in family participation in facility events
- Increase in special attention, affection, and supplemented services by families.

Implementing a family quality assurance program that aggressively recruits and serves the family as a client of the nursing home will increase the quality of family relationships and increase the quality of family/staff relations. Also, it is not costly to the facility, and will tap family resources to enrich the lives of the residents and the nursing home as a whole.

Chapter **16**

HOW CAN QUALITY ASSURANCE IMPROVE THE NURSING HOME'S ENVIRONMENT?

The delivery of quality care to nursing home residents begins with the identification of the residents' health and safety needs. Residents should feel secure in the facility as well as during trips into the community. State and federal laws governing the home's physical environment have been established to protect the safety of the residents and personnel in the facility. While these laws supply a sound foundation for safety, they do not take into account individual needs. The means of *identifying* these individual needs can be incorporated into the home's quality assurance program. Some suggested ways to *identify* individual safety needs are:

- Consult with residents and their families about safety issues. For example, if a resident is afraid of sleeping in a totally darkened room, make a note of this fear on the care plan and instruct the evening shift to turn on a night light at bedtime.
- Examine disruptive behavior to determine if the cause is rooted in fear. If, for example, a resident becomes combative while being fed, it may be due to a daily rotation in volunteers that does not allow the resident to recognize and establish a relationship with any one volunteer. Try to recruit volunteers who will work with the resident several days in succession so that a relationship can

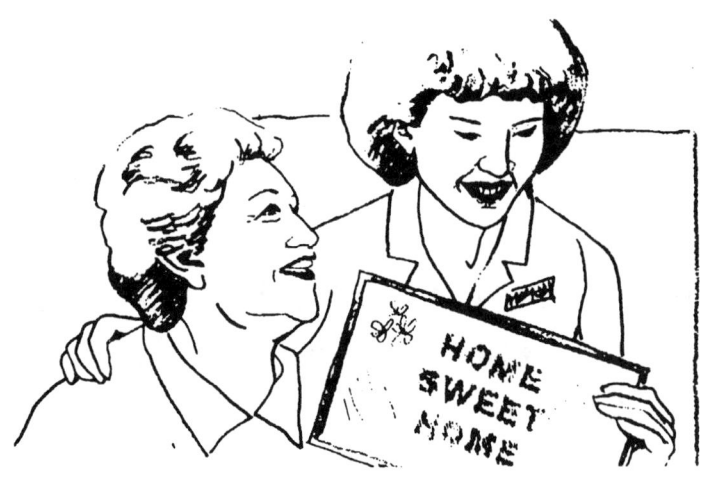

FIGURE 16.1 The facility is a resident's home.

become established before the resident must be fed by someone unfamiliar.
- Form a volunteer resident safety council whose responsibilities include detecting potential safety problems in the home, for example, slick spots on waxed floors or paper in ashtrays. The council may enjoy publishing a newsletter on safety for the other residents and staff.
- Bring in guest speakers such as firemen or policemen to give presentations on safety issues. Encourage residents and staff to ask questions and generate discussions after the presentations.

Identifying and meeting the health and safety needs of residents and staff is crucial to quality service in nursing homes. An effective quality assurance program can take improvement of the facility's physical environment one step further by creating an environment that is not only safe and functional but also cheerful and home-like. Because the nursing home exists for the benefit of residents and staff alike, a sense of home and family can be created by allowing reasonable participation by residents and staff in decisions concerning facility decor and purchases made for the home, such as plants, fishtanks, or magazine subscriptions (see Figure 16.1).

Some suggested ways to involve staff and residents in decisions concerning the facility's physical environment are:

- Form a resident decorating committee.
    - –They will be responsible for choosing new paint colors, placement of plants, pictures, posters, etc.
    - –Rotate members periodically so that everyone who wants to participate is able to.
- Display crafts made by residents and staff.
    - –Make a name card for each craft item so its maker is recognized.
    - –Ask if any of the makers are interested in giving a talk about their work; for example, residents and staff may enjoy hearing about how a quilt was made, the history of the pattern, etc.
- Devote a few minutes of staff meetings to inquire what would improve the environment for staff.
    - –Staff can vote for items to be bought for their benefit; for example, small appliances for the staff lounge.
    - –Reward implemented ideas for improvements with recognition such as telling about the ideas in the facility's newsletter or bulletin or displaying the person's picture on a wall along with a description of the idea.

Involving residents and staff in decisions concerning their nursing home promotes a sense of community within the facility, improves staff morale, makes residents feel "at home," and promotes a sense of ownership and control for everyone. Improving the facility's physical environment in small ways can improve the quality of life for the residents who have made the facility their home, especially when they are allowed to take part in decisions concerning their home.

Chapter 17

IS QUALITY ASSURANCE COST EFFECTIVE?

The quality of care can suffer significantly when nursing homes are forced to reduce the costs of service delivery. Deciding how and where to make budget decreases is an administrative task that will ultimately affect everyone in the facility. Budgetary decisions can be more easily made when there is a clear relationship between the facility's standards for excellence in care delivery and the costs associated with meeting those standards. Maximizing quality of service while minimizing the cost of service delivery is the goal of an efficient and effective budget.

To achieve an efficient and effective budget, administration needs some way of describing the relationship between cost and quality. As spending is reduced in the various departments, how is quality of service affected? Some suggestions for assessing the quality-cost relationship are:

- Examine resident make-up and variation in needs.
  - Can needs be met with fewer staff on certain shifts?
  - Which tasks require higher skill levels and which can be performed by employees with less experience or training? For example, how will quality be affected if an aide performs a task currently being done by an LPN?
- Consider the facility's hiring practices.
  - How is quality affected by hiring inexperienced employees at lower wages and providing inhouse training?

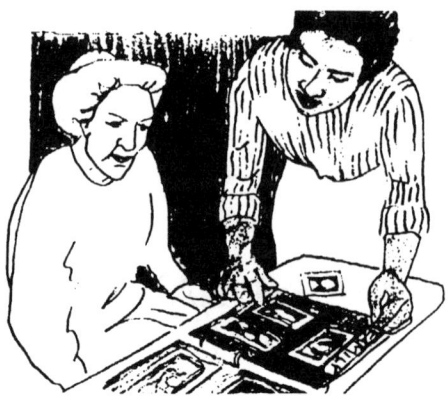

FIGURE 17.1 Volunteers are valuable resources.

  –Would there be advantages to raising wage rates for nurses in order to compete for the best nurses and reduce the possibility of high turnover?
  –Are there characteristics to common employees who have worked in the facility for the longest periods of time? Perhaps these are characteristics to look for in new employees that will reduce staff turnover.
- Assess your volunteer pool.
  –Does the community include many retired persons who might enjoy giving time to the nursing home and who are able to perform tasks currently being done by paid staff? (See Figure 17.1.)
  –Set up an incentive program for employees to recruit volunteers.
  –Are there merchants in the community who may be willing to provide services or goods in exchange for publicity?
- Examine buying practices.
  –Are there other facilities or institutions with which to join or form a cooperative buying group for bulk items?
  –What would be the cost advantages to buying fresh food in season as opposed to canned?
- Assess staffing patterns for efficiency.
  –Weekends are primary visiting times for families who may have questions, concerns, or information about their relatives that cannot be answered by weekend staff. Would there be

an advantage to having department heads available on weekends so that Mondays are not spent fielding telephone calls from family members?

The difficulty in making quality-cost tradeoff decisions is that while service costs are clearly defined and measurable, quality service is usually not. *Defining* achievable standards of excellence is, then, the first step in making cost-related decisions. *Planning* the means of achieving the standards is the second step. Maintaining the cost of the means within the predetermined cost parameters (implementation of the plan) is the task of the third step. Finally, an *evaluation* of the quality of service delivery in terms of cost must be done each time changes in staffing, procedures, or buying practices are made. From this cyclical pattern of *defining, planning, implementing,* and *evaluating,* quality-cost relationships will emerge so that quality service becomes measurable in terms of cost and cost becomes a direct function of the facility's performance standards.

Chapter 18

IS QUALITY ASSURANCE ATTAINABLE?

Quality assurance can be achieved in different ways depending upon the needs, the philosophy, and the perspective of the facility. Quality assurance can be achieved by a tightly structured program that uses checklists and heavy documentation procedures to measure the care being given and to make sure that staff members are meeting the expectations of the home. Quality assurance can also be achieved by a more informal program that relies on visual inspections by managers such as the administrator or the director of nursing. This type of program emphasizes vocal communication between management and staff to ensure that the care being delivered meets the facility's standards.

Although nursing home quality assurance programs can be very different, they share the common goal of providing quality care to the residents. The following are other properties of quality assurance that underlie all nursing home quality assurance programs.

- Quality assurance is a process designed by the facility's management to guarantee that each individual resident is receiving quality care.
- The quality assurance process is ongoing. This means that an effective quality assurance program is not a stop-and-start or

a one-time effort. A good quality assurance program is one that is being implemented at all times by all staff members.
- Quality assurance is closely tied to the facility's philosophy of providing quality care. Each facility has an idea of what constitutes quality care. Job standards are set and staff are expected to maintain them.
- Quality assurance is an important part of the field of long-term care and the field has certain ideas of what quality assurance should be like. Many of these ideas are the result of federal and state regulations for long-term care facilities. These governmental regulations are generally considered to set the minimal standards for acceptable levels of care. Regulations govern many areas affecting quality of care, including the facility's physical plant, the number and type of personnel, and infection control policies.
- Facilities can build upon the governmental regulations by raising expectations of what constitutes quality care above and beyond the minimal standards. This results in a facility's definition of quality assurance and definitions can vary widely from facility to facility.
- Quality assurance is continuity of care that cuts across all departments, meaning that everyone in the facility is responsible for the care of the residents. Housekeepers, the DON, the top administrator, nursing assistants, dietary aides, maintenance personnel, nurses, and anyone else employed by the home all contribute in some way to care of the residents and, therefore, contribute to quality assurance. Think about your job and how it contributes to care of the residents. How does it contribute to quality assurance in your facility?
- Quality assurance includes interaction among families, residents, and staff (see Figure 18.1). Quality assurance is more likely to be achieved when there is comfortable and open communication outside as well as inside the facility. Do you talk with family members as a part of your job? How does talking with families help you to help the residents? How does this contribute to your ideas about quality assurance?
- Quality assurance is a way of *identifying* and *solving* problems. What problems come up in your job and how are they solved? The problem solving methods of your facility are a very important part of your quality assurance program.

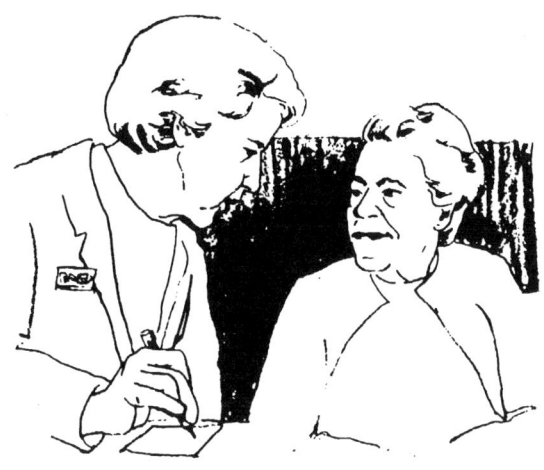

FIGURE 18.1 Quality assurance can be attained.

QUALITY ASSURANCE PROGRAMS

A quality assurance program in a nursing home is the means the facility uses to make sure the residents are being taken care of in a manner that meets the standards of the facility. The facility's quality assurance program is its system of *identifying* problems in the delivery of care, formulating *plans* to correct the problems, *implementing* the plans, and *evaluating* the outcome to determine if the plans were effective in eliminating or alleviating the problems.

There are two broad categories of quality assurance programs distinguished by the type and amount of documentation involved. The two types of programs, formal and informal, will be discussed and the variables a facility will want to consider in choosing the program most appropriate to its needs will be suggested.

Formal Quality Assurance Programs

Formal programs apply systematic procedures to measure the quality of care being delivered and require specific documentation as evidence that standards of care are being met. These procedures, along with the necessary documentation, are used by designated facility surveyors who are directly employed by the home or by the corporation if the home is corporate owned. Surveys are conducted at regular time intervals and may be as frequent as once per month or as infrequent as once per year. A single survey can last anywhere from 1 day to 3 months, depending upon its structure and purpose.

Although there can be a large degree of variation in quality assurance programs categorized as formal, all formal programs have some common characteristics. All depend upon checklists that determine what the surveyor is to look for or measure and how to do it.

Checklists consist of questions about the facility that the surveyor answers by marking the appropriate response on the checklist itself or by writing out an answer to the question. Here are some examples of questions that may appear on a checklist:

- Are bedrails up for all bedfast residents?
- Are all call buttons within reach of bedfast residents?
- How many non-bedfast residents are dressed in nightwear?

In addition to checklists, formal quality assurance programs use some sort of rating system to score or measure the facility's delivery of care by assigning values to questions that appear on the checklist. Nursing homes must then score a certain numbers of points to pass the inspection.

Formal quality assurance programs usually require the surveyors to document problems encountered in the facility and to make suggestions or help set up procedures for correcting the problems. Some formal programs also require documentation of outstanding features of a facility. Copies of the completed checklists and any additional documentation are distributed to the home's management personnel so the necessary improvements can be made and outstanding work recognized.

There is quite a bit of paperwork involved in formal quality assurance programs. To increase efficiency and reduce complications in the survey process, developers of the checklists should strive to cover all measureable aspects of nursing home services in as few questions as possible and with the simplest scoring or rating system appropriate to the questions. The simplest checklist would be a series of questions all answerable either "yes" or "no." Questions answered "yes" would receive a score of 1 and questions answered "no" would receive a score of 0. Facility management would then decide how many "points" a home must score to pass inspection.

Formal quality assurance programs may sound like a lot of work, but there are advantages to having a formal program. Well-constructed checklists make facility standards clear and deficiencies as well as strengths can be objectively measured by surveyors. Employees in each department know exactly what they must accomplish to pass inspection and are made aware of areas where they fall short of the standards. Plans of correction will be formulated and implemented within a specified period of time and the next inspection will determine if the plans were effective in eliminating the identified problems from the previous inspection. The next inspection will most likely reveal new problems and the formal process will begin again. This demonstrates how quality assurance is an ongoing and never-ending process in nursing homes committed to providing the best possible care.

Informal Quality Assurance Programs

Informal quality assurance programs are much less structured than formal programs. Informal programs rely more upon subjective problem identification and open communication between management and staff as the means of problem solving than upon written checklists, measuring and scoring techniques, and documentation.

Problems may be identified by the administrator as he or she makes daily rounds. The administrator will then call the problem to the attention of the appropriate supervisor and a solution will be sought on the spot, if possible, or at an arranged meeting of persons likely to be able to provide a solution. Problem identification, however, is not limited to the administrator or only to staff in management positions. All staff are encouraged to speak up if they notice problems or potential problems, and innovative ideas in service are encouraged and discussed. It is by means of verbal communication that facility standards are made known to employees, problems are identified, plans of correction are formulated and implemented, and effectiveness of the plans evaluated.

One advantage of an informal quality assurance program is that employees have the opportunity to contribute to procedures in the facility, thus developing feelings of pride and ownership in the home. A sense of pride and ownership will be reflected by more conscientious work habits, which will benefit the residents as well as the employees. Another advantage of informal programs is that the different perspectives of the employees can provide fresh ideas in approaches to care that can lead to greater effectiveness and efficiency in service as well as being cost beneficial to the facility.

To illustrate how the two different types of quality assurance programs can be used to solve a common problem in nursing homes, an example of a problem will be presented and solved using formal and informal quality assurance methods (summarized in Table 18.1, p. 93). The approaches are different, but the objectives of both types of programs are to:

1. *Identify* the problem
2. Formulate a *plan* to correct the problem
3. *Implement* the plan
4. *Evaluate* the plan for effectiveness in solving the problem.

Nursing Home #1: Problem Solving by Formal Methods

Once per month an aide from each of the facility's three floors is given the survey checklist used by the home's owner corporation to make annual inspections of its facilities. The aides switch floors and spend a day inspecting the floor just as the corporate inspectors would. This procedure for quality assurance teaches the aides facility standards of excellence and is instrumental in identifying and solving problems on a regular basis.

The aide assigned to survey the third floor records on her checklist that three residents are lying in wet beds at 3:20 p.m., just after the shift change. According to standards set by the corporation, all wet beds are to be changed by the respective employees at the end of their shift so that the new shift does not have to begin by changing wet beds. The surveying aide documents that three residents are lying in wet beds near the shift change. At the end of her inspection, she tallies the score according to instructions on the checklist. Because of the three wet beds, the floor does not score enough points to pass the inspection.

The checklists and additional documentation are presented to the DON by the aides the next morning. The DON meets with the charge nurse from the third floor to discuss the problem of the wet

Is Quality Assurance Attainable?

beds. The charge nurse is unaware of the problem so she schedules a meeting with the aides from the day shift to look for a cause and solution. The aides explain that because they are busy giving baths near the end of their shift, they are unable to complete other tasks, which include changing wet beds before the next shift arrives. So the problem *identified* by the survey as wet beds is caused by too much work to be done by too few aides in too little time.

TABLE 18.1 Comparisons of Formal and Informal Programs

QA Procedure	Formal QA Program	Informal QA Program
Problem identified	using survey checklist	through observation
Plan formulated	by management	by staff & management
Plan implemented	by staff	by staff
Plan evaluated	using survey checklist	through discussion

Formal QA Program Features	Informal QA Program Features
Service delivery monitored by surveyors using preprinted forms or checklists that quantify goal achievement or failure	Service delivery monitored by subjective observation of management
Plans for improving care delivery developed by managers	Plans for improving care delivery developed by managers in conjunction with staff
Relies upon objective measurement of data to determine effectiveness of implemented plans	Relies upon verbal communication between staff and management to determine effectiveness of implemented plans
Helps large facilities integrate employees of varying backgounds and values and who have little contact with one another	Helps maintain casual and family-like atmosphere in small facilities in which most of the employees have daily contact with one another
In-services usually scheduled and formally presented by department heads	In-services frequently presented on the spot by the managers who detect the problems

The charge nurse consults with the DON and they decide to try an earlier bath schedule so that the aides do not have so many tasks to complete near the end of their shift. Documentation of the *plan* is made and sent to the corporate office along with the original surveys used by the three aides. The new *plan* will be *implemented* for one month and then *evaluated* for effectiveness during the next survey.

The next month's third floor survey does not reveal any wet beds at times near the shift change so the plan of rescheduling the baths is determined to be successful and is continued as a quality assurance measure. The success of the plan is documented and sent to the corporate office along with the new surveys. The new bath schedule becomes a policy of the facility and is implemented by the other two floors as a routine procedure.

Nursing Home #2: Problem Solving by Informal Methods

In this nursing home, the administrator and the DON make daily rounds to monitor and evaluate care and to determine if all is going well. One afternoon around 3:20 they notice that three residents are lying in wet beds. Standards in this facility demand that all wet beds be changed near the end of each shift so that residents are not left lying in wet beds until aides from the next shift are able to change them.

The DON responds to the problem by asking an aide to change the beds immediately. She also makes a note to bring the incident up at the next staff meeting. Monthly meetings are held by the administrator for all department heads and for any other staff who may wish to attend. The purpose of these meetings is to inquire about problems or potential problems that anyone may be having and to develop ideas to solve or ward off those problems.

At the next monthly meeting the DON mentions the problem of residents lying in wet beds. An aide from the 3–11 shift remarks that wet beds are being left by the 7–3 shift who leave without completing duties which include changing all the wet beds.

The administrator prompts a discussion on what could be causing the occurrence of uncompleted work on the day shift. It is agreed that the evening shift has certain responsibilities that are being delayed because they must begin their shift by changing beds left unchanged by the day shift.

Through discussion, it is decided that the aides are having trouble completing their assigned tasks because they are busy giving baths near the end of the day shift. The problem is *identified* as too much work to be completed by too few aides in too little time.

The administrator asks for suggestions to eliminate the problem. An aide from the day shift suggests rescheduling the baths to an earlier time in the shift so that there is not so much to do at the end of the shift. The other aides in attendance agree that the *plan* sounds like an effective solution to the problem so the administrator asks the DON to reschedule baths in a way that is comfortable for the residents and efficient for the day shift. Staff agree to *implement* the plan for 2 weeks and then determine if the rescheduling of tasks helped the aides to complete their work by the end of the day shift.

During the 2-week trial period neither the administrator nor the DON notice any wet beds as they make their daily rounds. Residents are no longer complaining about wet beds, and there seems to be less tension during shift changes. At the end of the 2 weeks the administrator and the DON call a staff meeting to *evaluate* the plan. Feedback from the aides suggest that they are satisfied with the new bath schedule and desire to maintain it. Everyone agrees that the plan has been effective in solving the problem of too much work to be completed in too little time by too few aides.

The formal and the informal quality assurance program techniques in the above examples resulted in the same outcomes—a better quality of life for residents who were no longer left lying in wet beds and more efficient working procedures for staff. These are two goals that should be a part of the quality assurance program the facility chooses to adopt or develop.

HOW TO DEVELOP A QUALITY ASSURANCE PROGRAM

The first step in developing a quality assurance program that will be effective for your facility is to analyze the variables that make your facility unique. Some questions to be considered in the analysis:

1. How large is your facility in terms of staff; how are staff members alike and how are they different?
   - Is it small enough that management and staff have daily contact and problems can be discussed on the spot in a casual

manner, or is it so large that scheduled in-services are more effective for training staff?
- Are most of the employees recruited from the same area such that they have similar backgrounds and are familiar with the community? A small facility in which staff have similar backgrounds and values lends itself to easier communication than a large facility with staff of various backgrounds and value systems.

2. How large is your facility in terms of residents; how are residents alike and how are they different?
- Do you have many residents with widely differing medical and social disabilities requiring a diversity of staff skills or are you a small facility with residents requiring similar care so that your staff is interchangeable and each employee can work with any resident?
- Are your residents from the same general area such that they have similar backgrounds and values and communicate easily with one another, or are your residents from many different geographical locations, of widely varying economic status, and with obviously different value systems?

3. What are the characteristics of the facility?
- Are you located in a rural community where the pace is relaxed or is your facility in a busy urban area?
- Is your location such that community members have easy access to your facility or must they travel several miles to get there?
- How easy or difficult is it to transport residents outside the facility and into the community?

4. How will your choice of a quality assurance program affect staff morale?
- Will a tightly structured program using strict measuring techniques create unrest and feelings of competition among employees?
- Will a casual, loosely structured program result in staff not demanding as much of themselves as is required to achieve quality work?

Having answered these and other questions appropriate to your facility, you can decide whether a formal or an informal program will work best in your home to achieve your standards of quality care. After deciding on the type of program, the next step in its development is to determine what aspects of care will be monitored and how. Forms and/or checklists will be needed for formal programs and clear ideas of what to look for will need to be developed for informal programs.

Ways to translate facility standards into concrete and understandable working procedures for staff must be agreed upon by managers so that staff have a clear idea of what is expected of them and how to meet the expectations. Explain to staff what is being monitored, how it is being monitored, and why, so they have an understanding of how the quality assurance program works in relation to their own jobs.

When service delivery does not meet facility standards of excellence, correction procedures must be planned and implemented as quickly as possible. Determine general approaches to correction as a part of your quality assurance program, such as on-the-spot in-services when appropriate.

After deciding upon a formal or an informal program, developing monitoring tools and techniques, educating staff about the program and how it affects their jobs, and determining general approaches to problem correction, the final step in setting up a quality assurance program is to design evaluative methods for determining the success or failure of your program.

As you develop your own quality assurance program or if you decide to purchase a quality assurance package, you will want to keep in mind that a successful quality assurance program will:

- Promote ongoing quality care of residents
- Aid administrators, supervisors, and staff in identifying and solving problems
- Create a positive image of the facility as a home rather than an institution
- Reassure families that their relatives are being given the opportunity for a good quality of life
- Encourage members of the community to volunteer time and services to the facility as well as involve residents in activities outside the facility
- Promote a clean and safe physical environment
- Be cost efficient and effective
- Be compatible with the facility's mission statement
- Promote holistic care of the residents, which includes issues of self-esteem, self-respect, and independence.

PART III

PERSONNEL MANAGEMENT

INTRODUCTION

The need for nursing home care is progressing at a rapid rate within the United States. Along with this increase there is growing recognition that the care provided by nursing home facilities must maintain certain standards and quality. Unfortunately, the available resources for these facilities often do not complement the provision of quality care. Nursing home personnel are frequently underpaid, which means properly qualified personnel are difficult to recruit. Once recruited, management is constantly concerned whether they will be able to retain these employees.

The focus of this section is on issues confronted by management and on guidelines for recruiting and retaining qualified personnel. The intent is to provide a resource to nursing home administrators, owners, and staff in their continuing efforts to hire, train, and retrain staff in order to enhance the quality of care. Part III identifies and discusses pertinent issues related to managing personnel in nursing homes, including the management approach, advertising and recruiting, hiring and terminating, personnel records, job analyses and job descriptions, salaries and merit pay, performance appraisal, training and development, and staff morale and incentives. Although this section primarily pertains to nursing, the suggestions can be easily adapted and applied to all departments within nursing homes and other long-term care facilities.

Chapter 19

MANAGEMENT APPROACH

Nursing home owners, administrators, and department heads are ultimately responsible for the level of service and quality of resident care. Employees are resources used in providing services and implementing quality care. Employee management is the process of motivating and assuring that employees implement services and provide care for the home in accordance with set standards and practices. Effective employee management includes:

- Promoting values related to the quality of resident care and the working relationships of staff
- Setting examples for staff through management words and actions
- Structuring lines of authority and delegating responsibility
- Designing systems of accountability for quality care.

STATING THE VALUES

Having a defined philosophy and commitment to quality care is extremely important in any nursing home, since this sets the values and expectations for all employees. Typically, expressed values from exemplary nursing homes include commitment to:

- High quality of resident care
- Staff accountability for what they do and say in relation to residents and other staff
- Staff working together as a team
- Mutual respect among administration, staff, and residents
- Prompt attendance by staff to resident needs and requests
- Involvement of family and community in resident care.

These values are expressed by staff and are stressed in initial interviews with all applicants. They are further explored and assessed in performance evaluations. In staff meetings, in the community, and in other gatherings, the values and philosophy embraced by the home are frequently expressed. Typical statements include:

- Resident care is everything.
- You can tell the kind of home by the type of aides it has.
- The staff are the ones that make the home.
- Staff have the freedom to carry out their work.
- Management sets the example for staff.
- Daily feedback to staff on their performance is necessary.
- Provide immediate management intervention when deficiencies are observed.
- We train people to help each other.

SETTING THE EXAMPLE

The owner, administrator, and department heads set the example for employees through their actions. These actions include:

- Being intimately involved in the work of each staff member by making rounds to observe the quality of care being given and being involved in the teaching, training, and evaluation of staff
- Maintaining an open-door policy and discussing with staff any concern they want to address, including personal problems (see Figure 19.1)

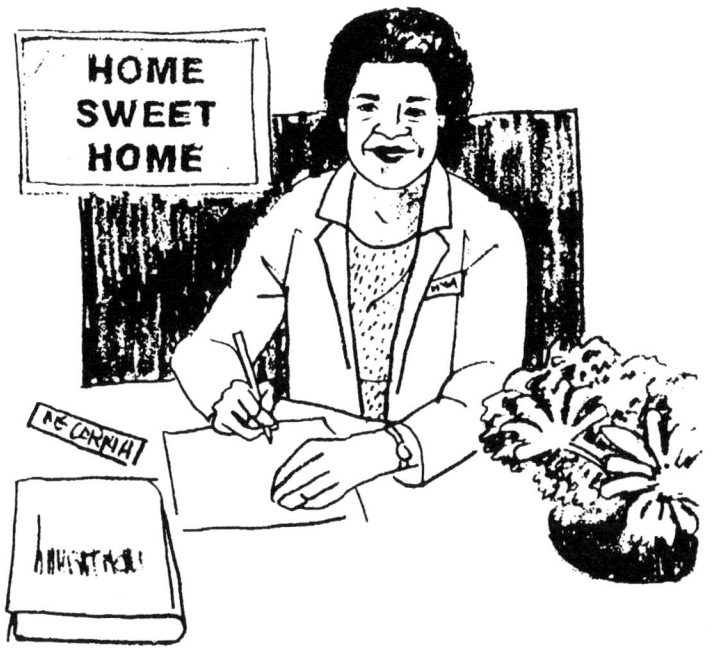

FIGURE 19.1 A concerned administrator readily interacts with residents and staff.

- Providing personal or financial assistance to staff (e.g., granting a small, interest-free loan to be taken out of the next paycheck)
- Relating well to the staff and seeking to learn something about the life of each person.

STRUCTURING AUTHORITY AND DELEGATING RESPONSIBILITY

While the administrator and the owner's involvement in hiring, firing, conducting performance evaluations, and scheduling varies from home to home, department heads are generally responsible for managing employees. The relationship among owner, administrator, and department head can be:

A consulting relationship in which these individuals give and get advice and direction from each other (e.g., the department head discusses an employee's performance with the administrator; the administrator discusses strategies of advertising with the owner).

An active relationship in which department heads and the administrators are jointly involved in personnel matters (e.g., the administrator and department heads jointly conduct performance evaluations, inspections, hire staff, schedule, and conduct in-service training sessions, etc.).

In nursing homes, organizational charts are important mechanisms for delineating work, defining responsibility, and assuring accountability. An organizational chart reflects the lines of authority and accountability within a home. In a chart, job categories (director of nursing, charge nurse, housekeeper, etc.) are listed with positions located higher in the chart having greater authority. Lower level positions are accountable to higher level positions and are connected by straight lines. Broken lines represent consulting relationships (see Figure 19.2).

STRUCTURING ACCOUNTABILITY

A job description states the specific responsibilities and duties assigned to each position. Each person in a position is accountable to a higher level position for the responsibilities stated in the job descriptions. However, in the operation of a nursing home, what is expected of each position changes depending upon the residents, physician's orders, etc. In order to maintain accountability and assure quality service, the following procedures are implemented:

- Systematic inspections of resident rooms, resident medical records, facility services (e g., kitchen, laundry, etc.).
- Performance appraisals of all staff to evaluate and discuss tasks, responsibilities, work quality, and quantity.

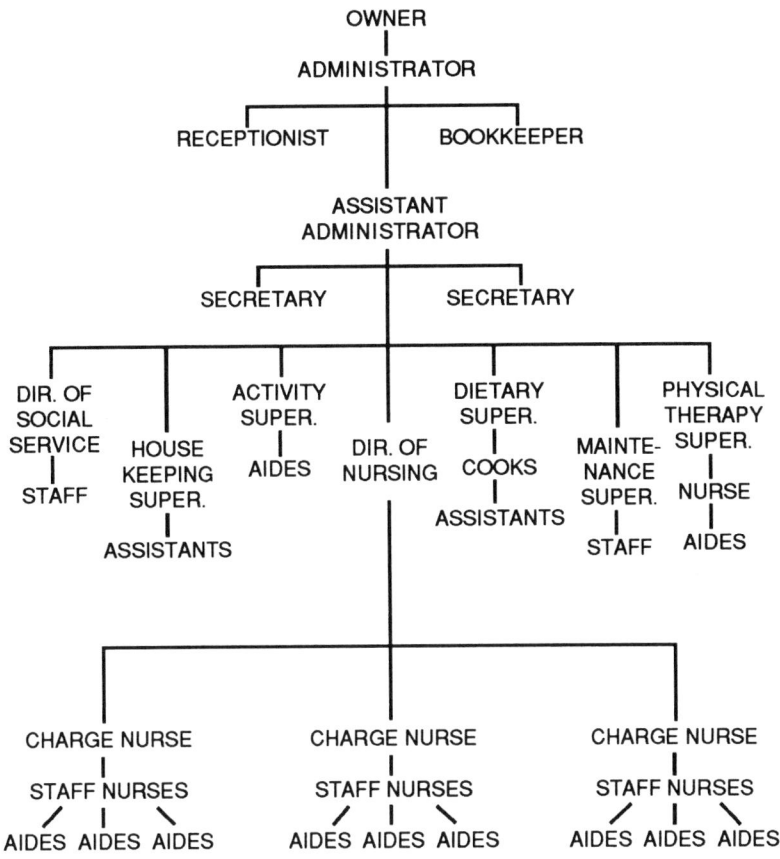

FIGURE 19.2 Sample Organizational Chart.

Rounds

Regularly scheduled rounds by the administrator, department heads, and supervisors insure that services meet an established level of care. Inspection rounds include an assessment of:

- Care of the residents (e.g., personal hygiene, hair, clean clothes, etc.)
- Compliance with orders (e.g., turning a resident in bed at certain times)
- Cleanliness of the rooms.

When an observed level of care, standard, or procedure is not what is expected:

1. Schedule a short, but immediate in-service with staff to discuss the expected standard of care, practice, or procedure.
2. Record the variation from the standard and place the concern on the agenda for the following in-service training session.
3. Request the responsible staff person to correct the deficiency immediately.

Chapter **20**

STAFF COMPOSITION AND RETENTION

The characteristics of staff in nursing homes are a reflection of the employment pool from which applicants are drawn as well as an expression of the management philosophy and the needs of the home. For example, staff employed in an urban area reflect different characteristics than the staff in a rural area; staff in a home for the developmentally disabled are different from staff in a home for elderly residents. The particular characteristics of a home's staff have implications for:

- The management approach
- Training and development
- Salary and merit pay systems.

The skills, abilities, background, personal needs, and status of employees determine the need for training, supervision, and support. When hiring, the capabilities of a prospective employee should be compatible with the needs and resources of the home. The following are characteristics to be considered in hiring.

Educational background: Staff with lower levels of education may require more supervision (especially when reading and writing skills are poor). Written orders and procedures may need to be discussed more fully with the staff and in-service training programs might need to be more specific in describing what is expected and how to perform the duties.

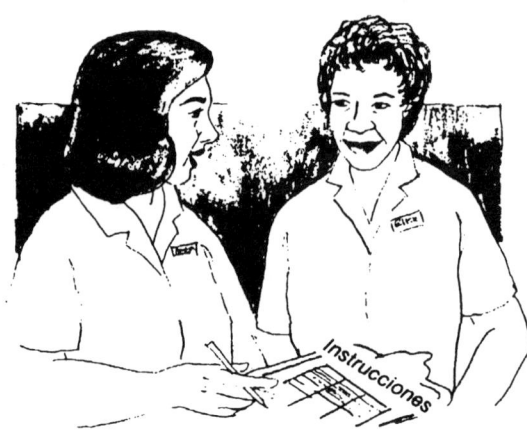

FIGURE 20.1 Job responsibilities and instructions need to be communicated in a way that staff can understand them.

Spoken language: An employee with a primary language other than English may need to have instructions in his/her native language (see Figure 20.1). For example, a Spanish-speaking housekeeper needs a job description and other written materials in Spanish. A bilingual staff person (e.g., supervisor) may be needed. Training will need to include more demonstration or "on-the-job" training than classroom teaching unless bilingual materials are available.

Household income: Staff should be encouraged to participate in on-going training efforts. Continuing education is essential to meet certification requirements. Staff from a lower income household would benefit greatly from financial assistance provided by the home for certification, continuing education, and training. An aide can be referred to certification programs that are subsidized through grants. Some certification programs offer tuition waivers to students who have a financial need.

Sex: Resident attitudes need to be considered in recruiting and assigning staff. Some residents want female aides and are uncomfortable with male aides, while other residents prefer male workers.

The use of part-time versus full-time staff reflects the management philosophy as well as the needs of the home. In homes for the developmentally disabled, where many residents may leave during the day to go to sheltered workshops or vocational training programs, part-time staff provide a cost effective way of serving the needs of residents in the evenings and on weekends. Part-time positions can be used to:

- Evaluate the performance of staff before they are offered the opportunity to move to full-time employment
- Meet the flexible work needs of some staff.

Chapter 21

ADVERTISING AND RECRUITING

The home's approach to recruiting staff can impact on the overall personnel costs by reducing the likelihood of turnover and retraining. Careful recruiting methods insure that the prospective employee meets the needs of the home and can effectively relate to other staff. When advertising, recruiting, and hiring, the Equal Employment and Affirmative Action guidelines must be followed.

EQUAL EMPLOYMENT OPPORTUNITY AND AFFIRMATIVE ACTION

1. Place the statement,"An Equal Opportunity Employer" in advertisements, job postings, and application materials.
2. Adopt written policies on Equal Employment Opportunity and Affirmative Action.
3. Post Equal Employment Opportunity and Affirmative Action policies in a visible and public place in the home.

RECRUITING STAFF

The issue of finding and attracting qualified staff is a concern of nursing homes. The basic methods of recruiting staff include:

- Referrals by current staff
- Referrals from area instructors of certified nurse's aide (CNA) programs
- Inquiries from newspaper ads.

Word of Mouth

A way of finding staff that is frequently used is through word of mouth. Employees who are aware of openings can recruit friends and others. Staff knowledge of the qualifications and integrity of potential employees serves as a resource to management Benefits of this method of recruitment include:

- The current staff person knows the needs of the home and believes the prospective employee will do a good job.
- The new employee will receive support while becoming orientated to the position.
- The referring employee assumes some responsibility for the new employee, thus "keeping an eye" on the individual.

This process of recruitment is formalized by offering staff a finder's fee for every employee they refer who is hired, is a good worker, and continues with the home for a minimum of 3 months. The finder's fee encourages staff referrals, while reducing the costs of advertising.

Certification Programs

Look for potential staff in certification programs sponsored by area vocational schools or community colleges. When the clinical part of the Certified Nurse's Aide (CNA) program is offered in the nursing home, staff develop a familiarity with the students. On staff recommendations, the best students can be offered employment. When the CNA program is not run through the home, the director of nursing or the administrator can request recommendations from the CNA trainer.

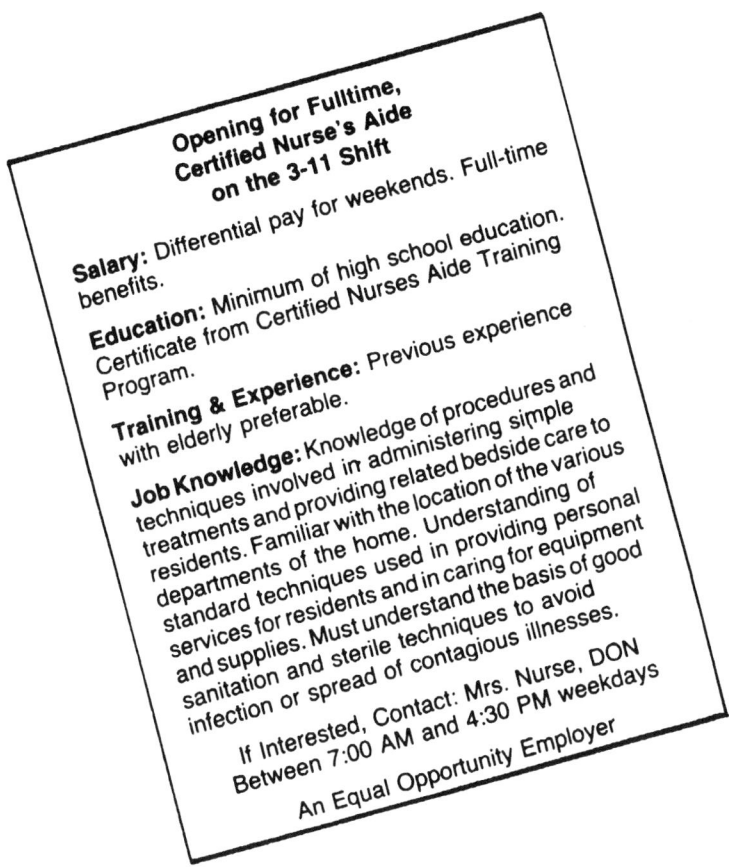

FIGURE 21.1   Sample Job Posting

Job Posting and Advertising

Job announcements are used to attract and recruit potential applicants for open positions. Announcements are posted internally and/or placed in newspapers or journals. A job announcement includes:

- Position title: e.g., nurse's aide, R.N., charge nurse, housekeeper, etc.

- Number of hours/days of the week worked e.g., 3–11 shift, full-time position; 7–3 shift on weekends, part-time position, etc.
- General responsibilities of the position: e.g., passing medications, working with residents, general maintenance, etc.
- Qualifications: e.g., certified nurse's assistant, high school education, 3 year's experience working with residents, etc. (See Figure 21.1.)
- Wages and benefits: e.g., starting salary $4.50/hr., salary and benefits are competitive, excellent benefit package, etc.
- How to apply: e.g., apply in person, call, or write to, etc.
- Name, address and/or telephone number of the home
- Contact person: e.g., call the director of nursing, call or write the personnel office, etc.

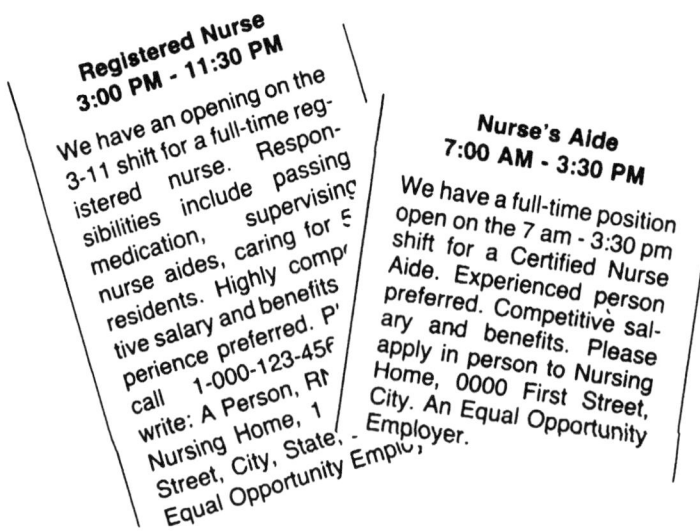

FIGURE 21.2 Sample Newspaper Advertisements

Internal Announcements

Open positions are posted and announced within the home. This gives employees the opportunity to consider transfers and promotions. Also, it motivates staff to consider additional training in order to qualify for such a position in the future.

Newspaper Advertisements

Job announcements can be placed in local newspapers to recruit applicants (see Figure 21.2). If the local labor pool is limited, place ads outside the local area.

Chapter 22

HIRING

Typically, in nursing homes, there is a high employee turnover rate. Adequate screening and well-conducted interviews identify employees who meet the needs of the home and others who may present problems. Careful hiring procedures can reduce the rate of turnover. The hiring process consists of the following steps:

1. Distributing and receiving applications
2. Conducting an initial screening of applicants
3. Interviewing screened applicants
4. Describing the job and responsibilities
5. Evaluating applicant interviews
6. Reference checks on promising applicants
7. Second interviews, if indicated
8. Final selection.

STEPS IN DISTRIBUTING AND RECEIVING APPLICATIONS

- Have applicants come to the home to fill out an application.
- Have a central person, such as the receptionist, office manager, etc., distribute and accept the application.

```
            Application for Nurse's Aide
            (An Equal Opportunity Employer)
  Name (last, first, middle) _____
  Address _____
  Phone _____ Emergency phone numbers _____
  Desired salary _____
  School where certification was received:
  Name of school _____ Date received _____
  Number of years of experience related to job (circle one)
  1 2 3 4 5 6 or more

                            Dates
  Previous    Address &     of Employment  Super-   Reasons for
  Employer    Phone         (from)  (to)   visor    Leaving
  _____
  _____

              Name &                Years
  Education   Location              Completed   Graduate
  Elementary     _____   _____    □Y □N
  High School    _____   _____    □Y □N
  College        _____   _____    □Y □N
  Special Training _____   _____    □Y □N

  Applicant's Signature_____ Date _____
```

FIGURE 22.1 Sample Employment Application

Application

The purpose of the application form is to provide the home with basic information on the applicant, including:

- Educational background
- Positions held
- Duration of previous positions
- Reasons for leaving previous employment
- Essential demographic information (e.g., birthdate, address, phone number, etc.). (See Figure 22.1).

The information on the application form is used to conduct the interview. Applicants are asked to explain any discrepancies or patterns occurring in the application (e.g., frequent moves, reasons for leaving previous employer, no nursing home experience, etc.).

STEPS IN INITIAL SCREENING OF APPLICANTS

1. Have a central person screen the applicant's general characteristics (e.g., appearance, motivation, politeness, etc.).
2. Refer those applicants who meet the home's expectations to the designated person for further screening or interviewing.
3. If a position is not open, inform the applicant that his/her application will be kept on file until an appropriate vacancy occurs.

INTERVIEWING SCREENED APPLICANTS

The administrator, department head, or both are involved in the actual interviewing and hiring process (see Figure 22.2). In nursing homes where the administrator assumes responsibility for interviewing and hiring, the employees will reflect the judgments and preferences of the administrator. (For example, if the administrator is aggressive, he/she might be more comfortable with passive employees, or the administrator may be biased toward older employees.) This has the advantage of providing internal consistency in the hiring process and in the selection of staff. Where department heads assume the responsibility for interviewing and hiring, the staff will reflect the department heads' judgments and preferences. This establishes accountability to the immediate supervisor from the onset of employment. When the administrator and the department head do the interviewing together, the advantages of both methods are combined. The disadvantage of involving both in the hiring is the time invested. Where it is not reasonable for the administrator to be involved, another department head can participate. When a department head position is being filled, the administrator interviews three to five candidates. Several interviews are

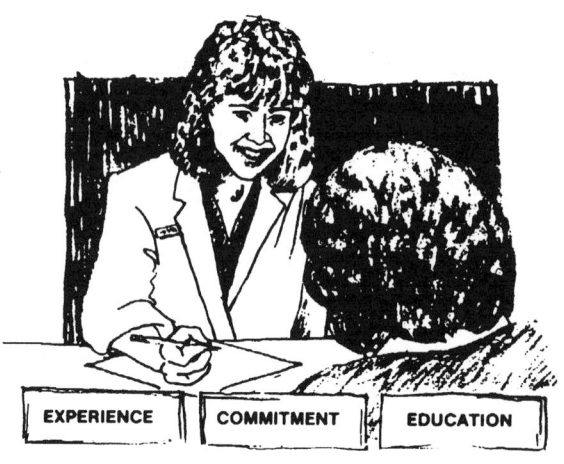

FIGURE 22.2 The personal interview is essential for selecting the proper person to fill a vacancy.

conducted with each candidate to narrow the number. If the home is part of a corporation, two finalists are recommended to the corporate regional manager, who makes the job offer in consultation with the administrator. If the home is not part of a corporation, the administrator, the owner, or board of directors makes the job offer.

Interview

The purpose of the employment interview is to gain information about the employee in the following areas:

- Dependability
- Responsibility
- Educational backgound
- Skills and abilities
- Commitment to nursing home care
- Attitudes toward elderly, authority, staff relationships
- Personal goals
- Desires in a job

- Way of relating to others (co-workers, residents, family members, etc.).

The following questions can provide information about these areas and will give the interviewer a good sense of the applicant as a prospective employee.

Interview Questions

- Why are you interested in nursing homes?
- How do you feel about the elderly?
- What are some of your personal goals?
- How would you work with someone who is confused?
- What do you think or feel about the home or place in which you previously worked?
- What was the length of notice you gave your previous employer?
- If I were to call the nursing home where you worked previously, what are they likely to tell me about you in relation to your attendance, personality, attitude towards work, and attitude towards residents?
- What is the most difficult thing you found about working in a nursing home?
- Why did you leave your last place of employment?
- What sorts of problems did you experience in your previous place of employment?
- If you join the staff, what contribution will you make?

Specific Questions to Nurse's Aides

- Why do you want to be a nurse's aide?
- What do you think is the nurse's aide's job?
- Describe your relationship with the director of nursing where you used to work.
- Do you have any concerns about working as a team member? What strengths would you bring to a team?
- What shifts do you prefer to work?

Applicant's Name _____ Date _____				
	Excellent	Good	Fair	Poor
Attitude of applicant	1	2	3	4
Appearance	1	2	3	4
Overall personality	1	2	3	4
Qualifications to do the work	1	2	3	4
Work history	1	2	3	4

Summary of strengths and weaknesses:

_____

Special training and skills relevant to the job:

_____

Recommendation: Hire   Hire/Caution   Do Not Hire
Availability for employment (starting date) _____
Interview conducted by _____ Date _____

FIGURE 22.3   Sample Interview Summary Form

Other Intuitive Judgments (Interviewer's Assessment)

- Does the applicant like himself/herself?
- Does the applicant have a positive attitude?
- Is the applicant stable?
- Does he/she seem comfortable in the interview?

See Figure 22.3 for an Interview Summary Form on which the interviewer's assessment can be noted.

Information Shared During the Interview

The interview is a time to discuss many issues. First, explain in detail what the job entails and, if possible, show the applicants the job while it is being performed. Other issues to discuss include:

Hiring

```
To _____          Title _____
Agency name _____     Address _____
Applicant's name _____   Address _____
Position applied for _____
I hearby authorize the release of all information requested.
Applicant's signature _____
```
Work Reference
```
Employed from ___ To ___ Position held _____
Would you rehire? Y  N  Reasons for leaving ___
```

	Excellent	Average	Below Average	N/A
Attendance	☐	☐	☐	☐
Appearance	☐	☐	☐	☐
Honesty	☐	☐	☐	☐
Judgment	☐	☐	☐	☐
Initiative	☐	☐	☐	☐

Rater's signature _____ Title _____

Educational Reference

Degree, course or certification _____ Date _____
Comments _____ Signature _____ Date _____

FIGURE 22.4 Sample Request for Reference.

- Salary and benefits
- Uniforms, appearance
- Work scheduling details
- Nature of the work
- Working as a team member
- Shift responsibilities
- Supervision of work
- Accountability for quality of resident care
- Union fees and dues, if applicable
- Training period
- Management philosophy
- Pay and merit system.

Reference Checks

The purpose of checking references is to get additional information about the employee's work habits, experience, skills, and ability. Check three references provided by the applicant. Due to a concern about being sued for giving poor references on previous employees, many employers provide information only about dates of employment and job responsibilities. In these situations, telephone contact can prove helpful. If a reference is not available by phone, send a "request for reference" form (see Figure 22.4). A helpful reference form has the following characteristics:

- It is standardized—all applicants complete the same form.
- It is signed by the employee, giving permission to release all information related to previous employment.
- It provides a self-addressed, stamped, return envelope.
- It provides a checklist for the previous employer to mark responses.
- It is confidential.

Chapter 23

PERSONNEL RECORDS

Personnel records comprise a written collection of employee information and work history with the home. These records serve as a convenient reference for management and as a source of documentation for Equal Employment Opportunity and Affirmative Action guidelines. Materials in the personnel files are to be signed by the employee. For non-English speaking employees, materials are translated into primary languages.

CONTENT OF PERSONNEL FILES

Basic information which is contained in an employee's personnel file includes:

- Yearly health exam form
- Orientation checklist
- Resident rights statement
- Application for employment
- Employee evaluation form
- Copy of W-4 tax form
- Emergency information sheet
- Responsibility of employees in fire situations
- Job description
- Copy of social security card
- Reference check form.

Information on work history which is contained in the employee's personnel file includes:

- Performance evaluations
- Warning, infraction reports
- Salary and merit records
- Certificates of attendance for
  a. State mandated in-services
  b. In-services, continuing education
- Records on leaves and paid holidays
- Special citations
  a. Employee of the month
  b. Special contributions
- Copies of certification and/or licensure.

CONFIDENTIALITY OF EMPLOYEE RECORDS

It is important to keep all employee records confidential. Keeping employee records confidential encourages trust between management and employees. Confidentiality encourages employees to can-

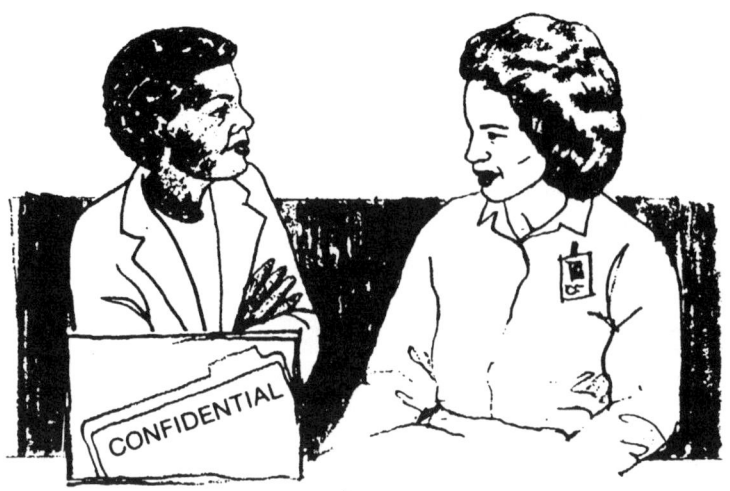

FIGURE 23.1 Personnel issues need to be discussed confidentially.

didly discuss performance concerns with their supervisor (e.g., an employee who has a poor performance evaluation will be more motivated to improve if he/she knows the results of the evaluation will not be shared throughout the home). In addition, confidentiality sets a standard of respect for individual privacy within the home. (See Figure 23.1.) To insure the confidentiality of personnel information, the following guidelines are suggested:

- Locate personnel records in a secure room in a locked file.
- Only designated personnel (e.g., administrator, department head, records secretary) may access personnel files.
- Control access of records by personnel through a specific person (e.g., records secretary).

Chapter 24

JOB ANALYSIS AND JOB DESCRIPTION

A job description is a written document outlining the general duties, responsibilities, and reporting requirements for each position within the home. Job descriptions are developed through a process of job analysis. A job analysis is a detailed assessment of what each job involves (e.g., tasks, responsibilities, authority, etc.). A systematic job analysis can:

- Highlight staff training and development needs
- Provide greater understanding of what staff are doing in their jobs
- Make clear the expectations for each position
- Form a basis for conducting the performance evaluation
- Create opportunities to develop new positions
- Yield job descriptions.

STEPS INVOLVED IN CONDUCTING JOB ANALYSIS

1. Questionnaire: Complete a job analysis questionnaire for each current or anticipated job (employee and/or supervisor, see Figure 24.2).
2. Evaluate the functions of each job and compare each job to all other jobs in the home, using the following criteria:

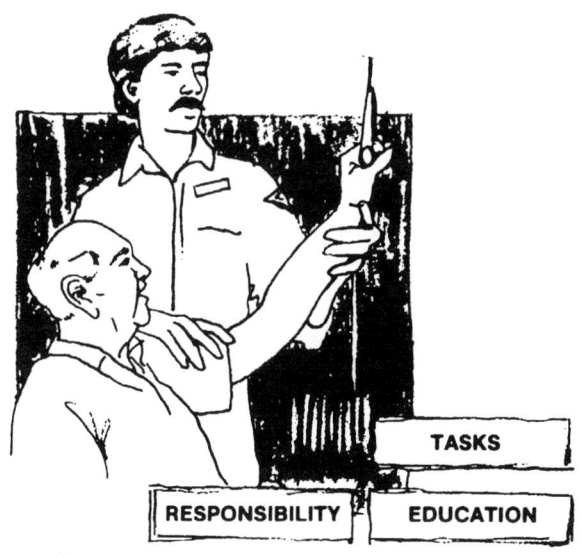

FIGURE 24.1 Each staff position involves different tasks and responsibilities.

- What are the specific tasks assigned to this position and how frequently are they performed? (See Figure 24.1.)
- What and how much special training is required to fulfill the responsibilities of this position?
- How important is this position to the home relative to all other positions?
- How much, and what kind of responsibility is required of this position relative to all other positions?
- What are the consequences of poor judgment in this position?
- How many people report to this position?
- How agreeable/disagreeable are the hours and working conditions associated with this position?
- How much freedom is there for independent decision making?
- To what extent does the incumbent of this position relate to the residents, community, other staff? How often? For what purpose?

3. Develop job descriptions: The evaluation of current and anticipated jobs provides the basis for reassigning responsibility, developing new jobs, or monitoring current jobs. A new job description is a summary of the findings and decisions from the job analysis (see Figures 24.3 and 24.4).

Job Analysis Questionnaire

Answer the following questions as they pertain to the specified job position.

Evaluator (name, title) _____

Position evaluated: _____

Description of Duties

1. What are the general purposes and objectives of the work?
2. What duties are performed in the usual course of the work?
3. What duties are performed only at stated periods, such as weekly, monthly, etc.?
4. What occasional duties are performed at irregular intervals?
5. Give one or two examples of characteristic issues or problems that the position may be required to resolve.
6. How many people are supervised by this position? (list job names and number of people directly reporting to the supervisor)
7. Who supervises this position? (name and title) Who else does this person supervise?
8. What type of guidance is received as to how the work is done and from whom?

Performance of Duties

9. What is the lowest grade of education that should be required of a person starting in this position?
10. Describe any applied training or special courses needed in order to perform the duties satisfactorily.
11. What special licenses or certifications are required for the position?

FIGURE 24.2 Sample Job Analysis Questionnaire

Skills

12. What past experience is necessary for a new employee to have in order to learn to perform the duties of this position? Name the kind of experience, where, and how it can be obtained, and the time required to secure it.

13. Having the above education and experience, what would a new employee have yet to learn and how long would it take the employee to obtain sufficient practice in doing the new work to reach satisfactory level?

14. In what lower position could an employee receive training for this position?

15. What types of in-service training are required to remain competent in this position?

16. For what higher position in the agency does this position train the employee?

17. What is the most difficult part of the job and why is it difficult?

Physical Effort

18. What machines or other equipment are used in the job?

19. Estimate what proportion of time is spent in: standing, sitting, moving, close visual work, operating equipment/machines, other.

20. What are the physical requirements for the proper performance of job duties? (e.g. strength, height, dexterity, etc.)

21. What makes this position unique from other positions within this organization or in other similar organizations?

22. List any other requirements not covered above and any personal qualifications and characteristics which you believe a candidate for this position should have.

FIGURE 24.2 Sample Job Analysis Questionnaire (*continued*)

Responsibility

23. What is the responsibility for money, securities, or other valuables?
24. How serious are any performance or judgment errors that are likely to be made during the normal course of duties. Give examples.
25. What is the nature and extent of responsibility for employees under your supervision?
26. What additional responsibilities does the position have?
27. What personal dealings with residents and public are there in performing the duties of this position?
28. Roughly, what proportion of time is spent in dealing with residents and public?
29. Describe the work relationship you have with other employees of the agency, not including supervisors and subordinates.
30. How much travel is required in this job?

Working Conditions

31. What are the usual working hours? Describe the shift work.
32. What are the disagreeable features of the job?

NOTE: In a job analysis, it is understood that each description will ultimately include "Other duties as assigned."

FIGURE 24.2 Sample Job Analysis Questionnaire (*continued*)

Nurse's Aide 7:00AM - 3:30PM
Qualifications

Education: A minimum of a grammar school education with a high school education or equivalent preferred. Certificate from Certified Nurse's Aide Training program preferred.

Training and Experience: Previous experience with elderly preferable.

Job Knowledge: Knowledge of procedures and techniques involved in administering simple treatments and providing related bedside care to residents. Must be familiar with the location of the various departments of the home. Understanding of standard techniques used in providing personal services for residents and in caring for equipment and supplies. Must understand the basis of good sanitation and sterile techniques to avoid infection or spread of contagious illnesses.

Working Environment: Work indoors in well-lighted and ventilated areas. May be exposed to communicable diseases. Possibility of strains due to moving residents.

Performance Requirements

Responsibility: Handling and caring for residents to ensure their safety and comfort. Adhering to instructions issued by nurse. Performing duties in accordance with the methods and techniques which conform to the home's standards of quality. Providing maximum resident-care service as directed. Maintaining good housekeeping standards within assigned duty areas.

Physical Demands: Good physical and mental health. Constant standing and walking during work periods. Turning, stooping, bending, stretching, and lifting to assist residents, make beds, move equipment, and perform other related tasks. Finger and hand dexterity to handle delicate instruments and other equipment. Visual and hearing acuity to detect changes in resident's condition.

Special Demands: Must have a genuine interest in geriatric nursing. Willingness to work with the realization that errors may have serious consequences for residents. Patience and tact in dealing with residents, their families, and visitors. Some initiative and judgment in recognizing

FIGURE 24.3 Sample Job Description

Nurse's Aide

symptoms indicating a resident's adverse reactions to treatments. Willingness to perform a variety of simple repetitive tasks, many of which involve unpleasant conditions. Rapidity and accuracy in preparing instruments and supplies for use within very limited periods of time. Work under close supervision.

Job Duties

1. Set up clean and dirty linen carts daily.
2. Review your assignment of residents and their plan of care, including your cleaning assignment, break assignment, and any special instructions.
3. Receive report from the staff nurse about your residents, such as:
   a) anything that is different or special you need to do for resident
   b) any new admissions
   c) any job assignments not included in the written assignment.
4. Make rounds to check all assigned residents. Be sure residents are prepared for breakfast. Face and hands are to be washed. Oral hygiene is done, toileting or diaper change is completed, and residents are set up for breakfast in bed, chair, or dining room.
5. Pass breakfast trays, seeing that each resident receives proper diet and that the meal is hot. Set up tray for eating, butter bread, open milk carton, etc. according to resident's needs. Note how much each resident eats for documentation on patient care record and advise nurse of any decreased intake.
6. Trays of residents requiring spoon feeding or partial assistance with actual feeding shall be served last.
7. Collect all meal trays and place on diet carts. Clean overbed tables. Position residents according to turning schedule as needed and document on the turning schedule as you complete each turn.
8. Give bed baths and showers as assigned daily, including shampoos and nail care. Record care done in the patient care record. Report to the nurse any bruises, cuts, scratches, rashes, or any change in the resident's skin condition.

FIGURE 24.3 Sample Job Description (*continued*)

Nurse's Aide

9. See that all residents are properly dressed and hair is combed neatly. Give priority to residents going into therapy. Apply urinary leg bags as ordered, use medical aseptic technique, cover large drainage bag tubing with a fresh sterile catheter cap and empty the bag of urine.
10. Complete room, make beds, and see that clothing is put away and table tops and dressers are clean. Put personal soiled clothes in dirty linen cart and throw it in laundry chute by 11am.
11. Place soiled diapers in plastic bags, close by knotting and discard in garbage chute.
12. Incontinent residents are to be checked every 2 hours and changed as needed. Assist continent residents in toileting as needed.
13. Check and toilet residents on bladder training at 8am, 10am, noon, and 2pm or according to the individual's care schedule. Document on the training schedule and the I&O sheet.
14. See that position of bedfast residents, those with restraints, and those at high risk of pressure sores is changed every 2 hours or more. Document turning schedules as each turn is completed.
15. Report any unusual symptoms to charge nurse such as pain, fever, body rash, personality change, or any change in the resident's condition whether physical, emotional, or psychological.
16. Pass fresh water to all residents able to take fluids by mouth. Assist and encourage residents to drink fluids frequently unless otherwise ordered.
17. Pass morning and afternoon nourishments as assigned.
18. Prepare residents for lunch. See that residents going to dining room are taken on time. Repeat procedure as for breakfast.
19. Assist residents out of dining room after meal. See that they are clean, neat, and comfortable. Assist those who require a nap to bed.

FIGURE 24.3 Sample Job Description (*continued*)

Nurse's Aide

20. Any units of discharged residents are to be cleaned by housekeeping and the bed made with fresh linens by the nurse's aide assigned to that room. Pack belongings as instructed by the charge nurse.

21. Assist in ambulating residents as requested by the Rehab Department or charge nurse. Do ROM and ADL on residents assigned to you according to sheets and as requested, and complete documentation.

22. Answer call lights promptly and courteously whether or not it is your assigned resident. Answer call lights for other staff when they are on break. They will do the same for you. Keep the call light within the resident's reach.

23. Assist with admissions, including settling the resident in the room and completing vital signs and the clothing list.

24. Complete documentation on I&O, B&B, V.S., Patient Care Record, and any other forms required.

25. Be sure safety restraints are on where needed. All restraints must be released at least every 2 hours and the resident repositioned and/or ROM done as appropriate for the type of restraint used.

26. Make last rounds by 2pm, changing diapers, toileting and turning residents as needed.

27. Clean off your linen carts and put them at the linen room for next shift.

28. Report to the charge nurses on the resident's condition and whether or not your assigned work was completed by 2:45pm.

I, _____ , have read the above job description and fully understand the conditions set forth therein, and if employed as a Nurse's Aide, I will perform these duties to the best of my knowledge and ability.

Date _____ Signature _____

FIGURE 24.3 Sample Job Description (*continued*)

Charge Nurse 3.00PM–11:00PM
Qualifications

Education: Registered nurse from a 3 or 4 year accredited program.

Training and Experience: Previous experience or training in gerontology or long-term care of elderly helpful.

Job Knowledge: Knowledge of general nursing theory and practice, including drugs, biological, physical, social, and medical sciences, and their application for better understanding of resident-care problems. Thorough knowledge of techniques and methods of resident-care.

Working Environment; Work in well-lighted and ventilated rooms. Subject to minor cuts from instruments and burns from sterilizing equipment. May be exposed to residents having communicable diseases. Possibility of strains due to moving residents or equipment or injury from irrational residents.

Performance Requirements

Responsibility: Direct supervision of nurse aides and LPNs. Dispensing medications. Maintaining quality care for residents on assigned floor or wing. Assure completion of floor assignments and duties.

Physical Demands: Good physical and mental health. Finger and hand dexterity to handle and manipulate instruments and equipment. Visual and aural acuity to detect changes in resident's condition.

Special Demands: Must have a genuine interest in geriatric nursing. Willingness to work with the realization that errors and incompetence may have serious consequences for residents. Understanding, patience, and tact in dealing with residents, their families, and visitors. Memory for details. Ability to maintain good working relationships among staff supervised. Initiative in identifying problems in resident care and maintaining resident care in conformance with recognized standards. Ability to make decisions.

Job Duties

1. Receive report from nurse going off duty. At this time, you should be made aware of any new residents'

FIGURE 24.4 Sample Job Description

Charge Nurse

orders, medications, or procedures that you are to be involved with and any IVs or tube feedings to be done.

2. Count narcotics with charge nurse going off duty.
3. The team leader should assign the aides their residents, showers to be given, residents to be fed, vitals to be done, cleaning jobs to be done, supper and breaks to be taken. Review nursing assistants' assignments for accuracy, practicality.
4. Provide a pertinent report to the CNAs following report from the off-going shift.
5. Attend in-service meetings as offered.
6. Make complete rounds, checking residents to see if there are any new acute problems and ascertaining up-to-date status of current problems.
7. Notify supervisor of any incident reports with residents, staff, or visitors; changes in residents' conditions, or prior to calling physician for any reason. Note all orders received.
8. Pass 5pm medications, always checking an order if you question anything, and sign for them on the med record. Record PRN meds when, how, why, effectiveness, result, and any meds not given and reason.
9. Supervise aides as they start to get residents up for supper, making sure they get to the bathroom first, if necessary, and cleaned PRN.
10. Take supper before or after the residents' meal; one nurse must be on the unit at all times.
11. Supervise evening meals and check the trays when they come up to see that meals are served while still warm. Also check trays to see that the resident gets the right diet. Supervise feeding to assure adequate nutrition for all. Help feed as needed.
12. Supervise aides giving showers making sure that they are being done properly, including shampoos and nail care as appropriate.
13. Supervise implementation of skin care, bowel/bladder, ADL, and accident/fall programs, including care given and the documentation of same.

FIGURE 24.4 Sample Job Description (*continued*)

Charge Nurse

14. After supper, check residents and rooms to see that the residents are clean and dry and the rooms are straightened to be ready for visitors.
15. During visiting hours, the nurse should be available to answer any questions or complaints from family members. If any major problems occur, refer them to the supervisor.
16. Review day shift admissions and complete as needed.
17. Admit new residents to unit, orienting them to the room and facility, doing all admission procedures, filling in charts, and ordering meds, supplies, and meals as per orders.
18. Supervise the passing of nourishments at 7pm, seeing that appropriate residents receive their supplements as ordered.
19. After visiting hours, make sure aides get their residents ready for bed, making sure they are clean, dry, and have had mouth care.
20. Do treatments as ordered.
21. Pass and sign for 9pm meds, checking residents to see if they need bowel meds or sleeping meds.
22. Do charting on residents, recording anything out of the ordinary on nursing notes, 24 hour report sheet, and required goal oriented charting. Monitor and supervise nursing assistants' documentation.
23. Make final reports on residents and rooms, also checking job assignments given to aides to make sure they are completed. Check residents with tubes for patency and restraints for proper application.
24. Give complete report to on-coming nurse.
25. Check narcotics and sedatives with on-coming nurse.

I, _____ , have read the above job description and fully understand the conditions set forth therein, and if employed as a Charge Nurse, I will perform these duties to the best of my knowledge and ability.

Date _____ Signature _____

FIGURE 24.3 Sample Job Description (*continued*)

Chapter 25

SALARIES AND MERIT PAY PLAN

Employees are a key in maintaining a quality home. A strong salary and merit pay system motivates employees to excel. To be effective salaries must be competitive within the local community. Having competitive salaries:

- Attracts more qualified staff
- Helps retain staff and reduce turnover
- Reduces costs (e.g., advertising, recruiting, hiring, training)
- Enhances employee morale.

SALARY SYSTEM

A comprehensive salary system is based on decisions and information gained through job analysis and salary surveys. Job analysis establishes the importance of each job relative to other jobs in the home, resulting in a job hierarchy. Salary surveys provide the prevailing costs to secure employees with the skill to carry out the responsibilities of a given job.

Steps to Develop a Comprehensive Salary System

1. Conduct a job analysis.
2. Conduct a salary survey.

3. Establish pay/salary ranges for each of the jobs within the home. Pay ranges extend from the salary paid to newly hired employees with no experience to the salary paid to long-time employees with considerable experience.
4. Establish salary increments or steps to reimburse newly hired employees for previous experience relevant to the job.

MERIT PAY SYSTEM

Incentive programs play an important role in strengthening morale, increasing job satisfaction, and improving quality work performance. Incentive programs can be either non-financial or financial. Non-financial programs include recognition by peers, administrators, and residents. This can be in the form of an "Employee of the Month" program, which may include a special parking place reserved for the employee, or special mention in the organizational newsletter in a section devoted to letters of thanks and appreciation to employees (see Figure 25.1.) Financial incentives come in the form of merit pay, benefits, career development programs, education and training, or paid child care.

The purpose of merit pay is to provide a financial incentive for employees to excel in the performance of their duties. Good work yields larger salary increases and poor work yields no increase. Merit systems are an essential part of strong salary systems.

A merit pay system can:

- Contribute to the overall quality of resident care
- Contribute to the performance of staff
- Increase the morale of the employees and the working environment in the home
- Determine the skill level and number of people who apply for open positions
- Contribute to the likelihood that qualified staff will stay
- Contribute to the job satisfaction of staff
- Recognize staff contributions to the home and residents
- Provide performance feedback to staff
- Provide incentives to staff.

Salaries and Merit Pay Plan

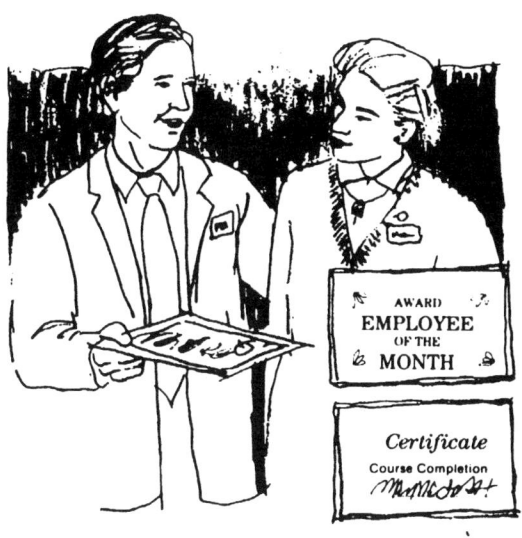

FIGURE 25.1 Staff must be recognized and rewarded for providing quality care.

An effective merit pay program needs to be linked to the performance appraisal system. The performance appraisal is an evaluation system used to determine salary and merit pay. Evaluations are based on the employee's performance. The rationale is that rewarding past performance will encourage quality performance in the future.

In manufacturing and production jobs, evaluations are often based on measures of discrete units of production for each employee. In other organizations the evaluation process focuses on the work group as a whole and rewards the group equally for their contribution to the objectives of the organization. In the human service sector the more common method of evaluation is by linking scores on the performance appraisal to salary increases. To be effective, merit pay systems need to be understood by employees, and the systems need to be viewed as equitable and fair by the employees.

Steps in Developing a Merit Pay System

1. Decide on the number of dollars available to be used for merit pay. The merit dollars are to be allocated to employees based on

ratings from their performance appraisals. For each rating a percentage rate of merit pay or given dollar amount is established. In homes with unions, negotiations are involved in setting these rates. Employees are rated as:

Outstanding: Performance exceeds all expectations for the position. Employee regularly proposes innovation in work; assumes leadership. Employee contributions of time and energy to the home are exceptional. Independent.

Competent: Strong contributions to the job. Employee usually meets the high end of expectations for the position. Demonstrates a solid and dependable work record. Independent most of the time.

Satisfactory: Average employee. Meets the general level of expectations for the position. Behavior may show variation. Generally needs supervision.

Unsatisfactory: Work is marginal. Employee demonstrates poor work habits and needs constant supervision. Probationary status pending.

2. Establish promotional increases with position changes or increased responsibilities (e.g., the advanced nurse's aide assumes responsibility for training new staff, assigning work, or monitoring team activities and an increase is awarded).

3. Establish increases for staff completing training or gaining new skills. For example, an aide who achieves CNA status or an RN who becomes certified in a restorative nursing program receives an increase.

4. Build other stages of employee activity into the salary and merit pay plan:
- Grant an increase when an employee changes from training to permanent status.
- Award an increase to an employee after the first 6 months of employment, then annually on the anniversary date of employment.

Merit Pay for Superior Performance

It is important that the employees understand that merit pay is given specifically for superior work performance. The criteria used for evaluating work performance has to be clear and applied uniformly. Otherwise, this can have an adverse effect on staff morale. Staff must understand that administration is not displaying favoritism in distributing merit pay. Further, they must know that these rewards are different from other bonuses given for holidays and birthdays.

Chapter 26

PERFORMANCE APPRAISAL

Performance appraisal is an evaluation of an employee's work. Conducted in an interview between the supervisor and employee, the appraisal compares what and how the employee performs with what is expected. Also, it highlights the standards and factors against which the employee's performance can be further evaluated (see Figure 26.1).

BENEFITS OF PERFORMANCE APPRAISAL

- Provides an understanding of the overall level of functioning of all staff in the facility, which is useful in deciding which departments, areas of performance, or skills need additional people or money
- Establishes a system of criteria to use in rewarding employees who consistently do good work
- Motivates employees through feedback from their supervisors
- Identifies skills and information gaps for staff, which is useful in planning in-service training
- Contributes information about the skills and abilities of current employees and is useful in predicting which employees to hire in the future
- Enhances employee morale

- Develops personal and professional goals for individual employees to assist in career planning and preparation for promotions
- Protects the home from lawsuits when employees are terminated for poor performance.

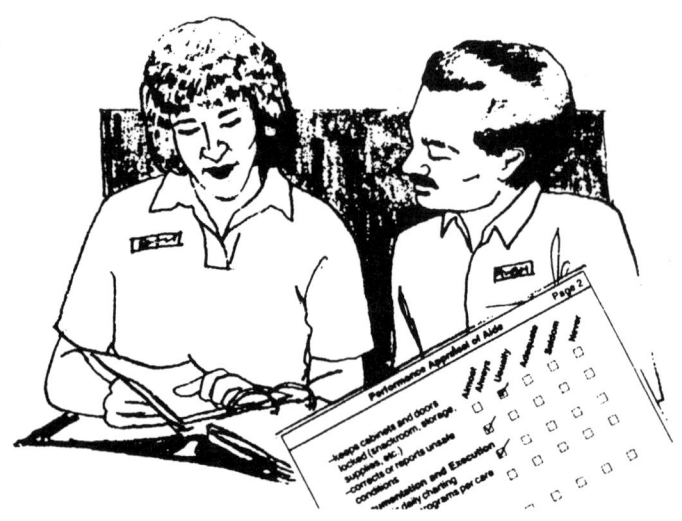

FIGURE 26.1 Work standards are translated into expectations for performance.

COMPONENTS OF PERFORMANCE APPRAISALS

An effective performance appraisal includes:

- Regularly scheduled interviews between the supervisor and the employee (e.g., every 6 months or every year)
- Specific statements about how, what, and when employees are expected to perform tasks (e.g., brush hair of residents, using their brush as stated in chart; demonstrate a pleasant attitude to residents by smiling, calling them by name, etc.)

- Goals for the employee (e.g., during the next 6 months have no more than 2 absences from work; attend 3 in-service training programs during the next 6 months; speak up at least 2 times in each team meeting; get residents up and involved in activities before 10:00 A.M. each day). These goals are agreed upon by the supervisor and employee and revised during each performance interview
- Assessments of how the employee does his/her work, as well as what results he/she achieves
- Employee feedback about working conditions, etc.

IMPLEMENTING A PERFORMANCE APPRAISAL

Different types of performance appraisals are:

Supervisory appraisals: supervisor and employee meet to discuss performance (see Figure 26.2).

Self appraisal: employee evaluates his/her own performance.

Peer appraisals: employees on the same team or same job evaluate each other.

Subordinate appraisals: employees evaluate their supervisors.

Resident appraisals: residents evaluate employees.

In implementing performance appraisals, one needs to:

- State what tasks are to be measured.
- Indicate how to improve what is done.
- Recommend or provide training and instruction.
- Be aware of judgments involving work behavior, personal feelings about the worker, and knowledge and evaluation of performance on the job.
- Maintain an interpersonal, problem-solving focus.
- Avoid talking only about "good" behaviors.

STEPS IN CONDUCTING A SUPERVISORY APPRAISAL

1. Employee and supervisor independently complete an evaluation of the employee's performance.
2. Employee and supervisor meet in a quiet and confidential atmosphere.
3. Supervisor begins by reviewing the findings of the last performance evaluation or current job description.
4. Supervisor discusses the good behaviors, abilities, and contributions of the staff person (e.g., comments from other staff and residents, attendance record, specific behaviors, leadership, etc.).
5. Employees comment and discuss their contributions and strengths.
6. Employees comment and discuss their weaknesses, issues, concerns, and problems in performance.
7. Supervisor adds or deletes from employee comments.
8. Employee and supervisor discuss working conditions, pay, staff relationships, etc.
9. Supervisor and employee agree upon new goals.

Performance Appraisal of Aide

Appearance and Conduct	Almost Always	Usually	Adequate	Seldom	Never
—uniform neat and clean, dresses neatly, good body hygiene	☐	☐	☐	☐	☐
—cooperates with peers	☐	☐	☐	☐	☐
—cooperates with supervisors	☐	☐	☐	☐	☐
—accepts corrections and is willing to improve	☐	☐	☐	☐	☐
—completes assigned tasks	☐	☐	☐	☐	☐
—enthusiastic toward resident care	☐	☐	☐	☐	☐
—respects resident's privacy	☐	☐	☐	☐	☐
—interacts appropriately with residents' significant others	☐	☐	☐	☐	☐
Dependability					
—reports to work on time	☐	☐	☐	☐	☐
—reports to work per schedule	☐	☐	☐	☐	☐
—assignments are followed through on a timely basis	☐	☐	☐	☐	☐
Quality of Care					
—resident rooms and work areas kept clean and neat	☐	☐	☐	☐	☐
—attends to residents' needs (feeding & elimination)	☐	☐	☐	☐	☐
—grooms residents appropriately (teeth brushed, shaved, hands and face washed and clean)	☐	☐	☐	☐	☐
—interacts in a polite way with the residents	☐	☐	☐	☐	☐
Safety					
—safely handles equipment used (wheelchairs locked during transfer, restraints on, etc.)	☐	☐	☐	☐	☐
—consistently uses infection control (hand washing, linen care, etc.)	☐	☐	☐	☐	☐

FIGURE 26.2 Sample Performance Appraisal

Performance Appraisal of Aide

	Almost Always	Usually	Adequate	Seldom	Never
—keeps cabinets and doors locked (snackroom, storage, supplies, etc.)	☐	☐	☐	☐	☐
—corrects or reports unsafe conditions	☐	☐	☐	☐	☐

Documentation and Execution

	Almost Always	Usually	Adequate	Seldom	Never
—records daily charting	☐	☐	☐	☐	☐
—carries out programs per care plan objectives	☐	☐	☐	☐	☐

Other Items

	Almost Always	Usually	Adequate	Seldom	Never
—attends staff meetings and in-services regularly	☐	☐	☐	☐	☐
—ability to establish working relationship with fellow employees and residents' significant others	☐	☐	☐	☐	☐

Overall Evaluation
___ Outstanding
___ Very Good
___ Satisfactory
___ Needs Improvement
___ Unsatisfactory

Comments

Comment on employee's major strengths, developments achieved since the last appraisal.

If overall evaluation is "Needs Improvement" or "Unsatisfactory," list steps employee is to undertake to continue employment.

Employee's comments on appraisal:

Prepared by (supervisor's signature) _____

Approved by (Administrator or DON) _____

This appraisal was discussed with me:

(employee's signature) _____ Date _____

FIGURE 26.2 Sample Performance Appraisal (*continued*)

Chapter 27

TRAINING AND DEVELOPMENT

The purpose of staff training and development is to ensure quality care for residents. Staff training is concerned with staff learning what is expected and acquiring skills needed to meet the expectations. Staff development is concerned with staff's emotional, professional, and career development. Generally, staff training and development are a part of a systematic staff training and development program (see Figure 27.1).

BENEFITS OF ORIENTATION, TRAINING, AND STAFF DEVELOPMENT

- Develops the necessary skills for staff who are hired with marginal skill levels (e.g., a new employee can be trained to perform at the level expected, even without prior training or experience)
- Keeps staff current on new developments in the field (e.g., new techniques and approaches to resident care can be integrated into staff performance through use of in-service)
- Addresses deficiencies in performance of staff (e.g., when a common problem is identified in the performance of staff, the problem is addressed in an in-service)
- Meets state mandated requirements for hours and types of training

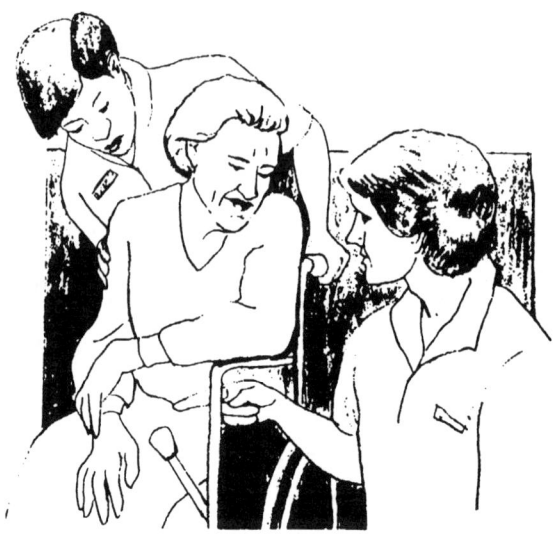

FIGURE 27.1 Systematic staff training is essential to ensure quality care of residents.

- Enhances staff morale and motivation (when employee knows what is expected and is trained on how to do what is expected, his/her willingness to work increases)
- Develops a pool of trained staff (e.g., staff trained by the home and supported for promotion into higher level positions)
- Improves retention of staff (e.g., a nurse's aide may want to become a licensed or registered nurse. If this person is a valuable employee to the organization, providing additional support for his/her training and development will be an investment, resulting in retention of a valuable employee).

ELEMENTS OF COMPREHENSIVE STAFF TRAINING AND DEVELOPMENT PROGRAM

- Assessment of needs for certain skill levels based on the home's goals and objectives
- Orientation

- Assessment of in-service training needs
- Performance appraisals
- Career assessments of staff
- Evaluation

STEPS IN DEVELOPING A COMPREHENSIVE TRAINING AND DEVELOPMENT PROGRAM

1. Assessment of the home's goals and objectives
2. Orientation
3. Assessment of in-service training needs
4. Conducting in-service training
5. Employee development and training

Assessment of the Home's Goals and Objectives

This assessment provides the basis for structuring a systematic training and development program. Examples of the questions that need to be included in a home's assessment of its goals and objectives include:

- Who are the residents?
- What are the particular needs of the residents?
- Is the home considering expansion?
- Does the home want to hire and promote from within?

Orientation

Immediately after hiring, an employee is provided an orientation to the home and the job. Orientation reduces employee stress and helps the newly hired to adjust to the job. Topics covered in an orientation include:

- Corporate and/or home policies
- Job description
- Employee benefits

- Employee ethics
- Philosophy of management
- History of the home
- Authority structure
- Rules of the home
- Disaster and fire policies
- Employee handbook

Orientation of new employees can occur in several ways:

- Supervisor meets with employee to discuss topics and demonstrate procedures.
- New employees are hired at specific times (e.g., once a week/month). Orientation sessions are conducted by department heads, supervisors, and/or administrator.
- New employees are assigned to the staff person who is leaving or are assigned to high-level staff. The assignment can range from several hours in the case of a secretary, to several days in the case of nursing personnel.
- Personnel from other homes or corporate offices may provide orientation and training.

Upon completion of orientation, the newly hired employee is evaluated using a skills checklist (see Figure 27.2). This evaluation assures that the employee has acquired the basic skills to begin employment. If deficiencies are noted, then additional training is needed.

Assessment of In-service Training Needs

The purpose of this assessment is to ensure that the training offered meets the needs of the home, staff, and residents. This can be accomplished in several ways:

Performance appraisals: During the performance interviews, problems in employee skills or understanding are identified.

Rounds or inspections of facility: During daily rounds or inspections of the home, deficiencies are noted (e.g., corners of the rooms are not kept clean; staff are having trouble reading charts; dirty laundry is on the floor, etc.).

Nurse's Aide: Orientation Skills Checklist*

Hand washing _____	Range of motion _____
Bed making _____	active _____
Bed bath _____	passive _____
Partial bath _____	assisted active _____
Shower _____	Clothing care _____
Hair washing _____	Serving trays _____
Hair combing _____	Set up resident for meals _____
Oral hygiene _____	Feeding _____
Denture care _____	Tube feeding _____
Skin care _____	alarm on pump _____
Nail care _____	taping tube _____
Dressing _____	trouble signs _____
Shaving _____	Types of diet _____
Bed pan & urinal _____	Temperature _____
placement _____	oral _____
disposal _____	rectal _____
Bowel & bladder training _____	Pulse _____
Intake & output _____	Respirations _____
Peri care _____	Blood pressure _____
Catheter care _____	Thermometer care _____
trouble signs _____	Urine spec. collection _____
tubing placement _____	Ice bags _____
bag placement _____	Water bottle _____
emptying _____	Chair scale _____
Linens _____	Restraints _____
use of _____	indications _____
care of _____	application of vest _____
cart set up _____	application of wrists _____
Positioning _____	Clinitest _____
decubitus prevention _____	Care of dying resident _____
turn schedule _____	signs of impending death _____
pillow placement _____	comfort measures _____
Transfers _____	Care of deceased _____
lift _____	Admissions _____
pivot _____	Discharges _____
walker _____	Transfers _____

Comments _____

Supervisor
signature _____   Employee
signature _____   Date _____

FIGURE 27.2 Sample Skills Checklist

*Form obtained from Lake Bluff Health Care Center

Staff meetings: Employees are asked: "What topics or concerns would you like addressed in an in-service training session'?" or "In what areas do you want to increase your skills?"

State mandated in-services: (Requirements as outlined in Illinois Administrative Code, Chapter I, 300.650(b)(3), 300.610(c)(2), Federal Regulations.) Employees shall attend in-service training programs covering each of the following topics related to their assigned duties, at least annually, and written records of program content for each session and employee attending is kept on file:
- Physician services
- Emergency services
- Personal care and nursing services
- Restorative services
- Activity services
- Pharmaceutical services
- Dietary services
- Social services
- Dental services
- Clinical records
- Diagnostic services, including lab and X-ray
- Prevention and control of infection
- Fire prevention and safety
- Confidentiality of resident information
- Preservation of resident dignity, including privacy, personal, and property rights

Required in-services also include:

- Material regarding the home's policies, skill training and ongoing education carried out to enable all staff to perform their duties effectively
- Material concerning prevention and treatment of decubitus ulcers (bed sores)
- Material on the effects of diet in treatment of various diseases or medical conditions and the importance of laboratory test results in determining therapeutic diets
- Presentation by advisory dentist or dental hygienist, pharmacist, and dietitian.

Management goals: New procedures or techniques (e.g., changing from rotating to permanent assignment, new techniques for docu-

menting care plan information, etc.) and personnel issues identified by management are incorporated into training. Topics include:
- Time management
- Stress management
- Self-concept
- Motivation
- Teaching skills
- Interpersonal communication skills
- Dealing with supervisors
- Dealing with difficult residents
- Aging issues
- Death and dying issues
- Mental health

Conducting In-service Training

Once the training needs are assessed and the value of the proposed training is determined, then training programs are designed and implemented.

Available resources: The resources available for designing and conducting in-service training programs are numerous, including:

- Staff resources: Current staff with the knowledge and skills in resident care, medications, handling behavioral problems, etc., can provide in-services. Using staff resources serves to recognize staff abilities; thus, increasing morale and reducing costs.
- Audio-visual resources: Universities and community colleges have catalogues of available resources covering numerous topics and procedures.
- External consultants and resources: Personnel are available in the community for conducting in-services. In areas of team building, conflict resolution, supervisory training, etc., external consultants are a safe, cost-effective resource.

Scheduling: The frequency and timing of in-service training depend on the needs of the home and the staff's quality of work (e.g., number of staff, turnover, nature of procedural changes, fiscal limitations, state mandates, etc.). In addition, the frequency and timing of in-services also depend on the issue needing to be addressed.

- Spontaneous in-services: Observed gaps in staff's current level of performance can be addressed through short, immediately-scheduled in-services. (E.g., while conducting inspection rounds, a nursing supervisor notices that residents have not been adequately groomed. An immediate in-service lasting 10 minutes is scheduled to confront the concern and discuss ways to handle the "problem".)
- Flexible in-services: With staff on three shifts, in-services need to be conveniently available to all staff. This can be accomplished through offering the session more than once and on different shifts, by videotaping the in-service for use on other shifts, or by reimbursing staff for attending during off hours.
- Structured in-services: In-services can be scheduled once a month at designated times, with tentative topics planned.

Evaluation of in-service training: Upon completion of the training program, an evaluation is helpful in assessing its effectiveness. Feedback from trainees can be integrated into the training materials to strengthen future in-services.

Employee Development and Training

A commitment to long-term employee growth and development can increase the retention of key staff. Employees seeking further training can be assets in the future. Options for supporting employee development include:

Scholarship/tuition reimbursement: An employee applies for tuition reimbursement from the home for a course of study in an area that will benefit the home or prepare the employee for an advanced position in the home. The employee has been employed for a minimum of one year and maintains a "C" or better grade in the course. The home determines a maximum amount they will pay to one employee in one year's period.

Registration reimbursement: The employee requests reimbursement for registration to attend a special training program, workshop, or conference. Reimbursement is granted on an individual employee basis.

Chapter **28**

STAFF MORALE AND INCENTIVE PLANS

In a nursing home, high or good staff morale is essential to maintaining a staff willing to be productive, committed to quality, and able to handle issues within the daily work activities. Morale is directly related to staff retention, turnover, and daily work attendance. The behavior of management and supervisory personnel in a home is a primary determinant of the staff morale within the home. A sensitivity to the individual staff person by his/her immediate supervisor opens the door to a collaborative relationship between the two. In a busy work environment it is difficult always to recognize the value of the contributions of staff. In these situations structured activities or celebrations recognizing groups of staff can let them know how important their services are to residents. In addition, recognition of individual staff by administration can contribute to overall morale of the home.

STRUCTURED INCENTIVES AND RECOGNITION

Staff parties: Holiday celebrations and annual staff picnics can be scheduled in the home. Remember that parties located away from the home preclude attendance by working staff. Prepare additional food, have food catered, or offer potluck. Award door prizes (e.g., certificates for gas, new uniforms, a grocery voucher). Give small gifts to each staff person (e.g., a pin, flowers, a bonus).

Annual nurses recognition day/week: Place posters on walls honoring staff. Give flowers to staff. Offer a free meal or potluck.

Employee of the month: An employee of the month can be selected by management or by the residents. Provide employee with private parking, give a corsage, display his/her picture, publish an article about the person in the home's newsletter, place the employee's name on a plaque, or give the employee a bonus.

Mother's Day/Father's Day and birthdays: Provide a corsage, give the day off.

Employment anniversary: Give flowers, special name tag.

In-services: Provide special treats, pins, certificates of attendance.

INTERPERSONAL RECOGNITION AND INCENTIVES

- Comment to staff about their appearance (e.g., hair looks nice, uniform unusually bright, seem chipper today).
- Look staff in the eye and recognize them by name when conducting rounds or walking around the home.
- Know about something that is happening in each employee's life.
- Tell staff they are doing a good job.
- Let staff know management is human by sharing personal stories.
- Demonstrate a concern about the employee's future by visiting with each employee once a year about their employment future.
- Write happy faces on pay checks.
- Work with staff on the floor.

ORGANIZATIONAL INCENTIVES AND RECOGNITION

- Provide staff with a lounge of their own. On special occasions or with gifts, purchase equipment for their use (e.g., a microwave, posters, a refrigerator).

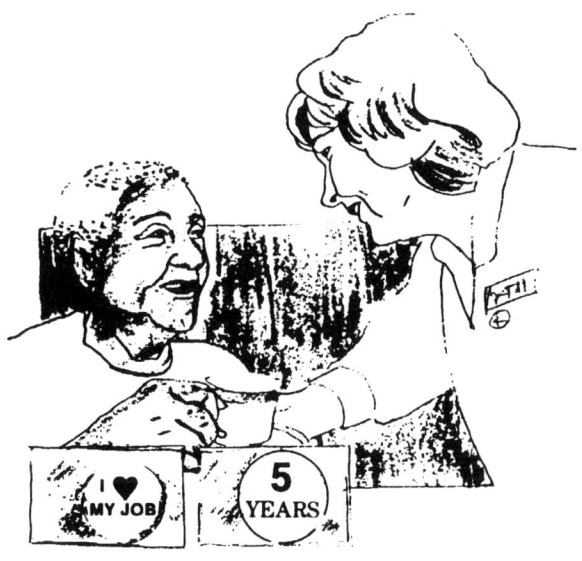

FIGURE 28.1 Satisfied employees stay with their employer and contribute more to their jobs.

- Provide staff with free or reduced cost meals. Such incentives may be tied to being on call over lunch periods.
- Offer small interest free loans to staff and allow repayment through payroll deductions over an agreed upon period of time.
- Give each staff person every other weekend off.
- If staff do not miss any time between Thanksgiving and Christmas give them a day off or a bonus.
- Provide bonuses for constructive employee suggestions.
- Respond in writing to all employee suggestions which result in improvement in the home.
- Provide benefit options for employees to choose.
- Provide health insurance.
- Offer tuition reimbursement for employees who submit requests to study in an area of importance to the home.
- Provide bonuses and recognition for excessive overtime.
- Develop opportunities for advancement and additional training.

- Offer to reimburse a part or all of the cost for obtaining certification. This can be contingent on longevity with the home. The nursing home may provide a loan to a staff member to obtain training with a portion of the loan written off for every month the employee continues to work.

Chapter 29

EMPLOYEE BENEFITS

A BENEFITS PROGRAM

Employee benefits are services offered by the home that promote the health, safety, and welfare of the staff. A benefit program has the following advantages:

- Staff retainment
- Enhancement of staff commitment
- Improved staff morale
- Rewards for longevity

A comprehensive benefit package serves the particular needs of staff as well as the needs and resources of the home. Generally, employee benefits are categorized in the following areas:

Insurance: Protecting the health, welfare, and fiscal resources of employees and their families (e.g., health, dental, life, disability, etc.).

Service options: Providing for the employees' convenience in time and financial resources (e.g., free meals, staff-physician health examinations, credit union, child care provisions, etc.).

Longevity: Rewarding employees for length of time with the home (e.g., sick leave, vacations, continuing education, leaves, etc.).

ELIGIBILITY

The eligibility of employees to participate in the home's benefit program is related to the following factors:

- Length of time employed with the home
- Number of hours worked per week
- Employment status (e. g., part-time, full-time).

ACTUAL BENEFITS

Possible employee benefits include:

- Vacations
- Shift differential
- Weekend differential
- Funeral leave
- Health insurance
- Tax exempt annuity program/retirement
- Credit union membership and benefits
- Paid in-service training
- Perfect attendance (day off)
- Birthday and Christmas gifts
- Employee discounts (meal tickets, prescriptions, child day-care)
- Overtime (1½) pay if work on holidays
- Sick leave
- Stock option purchase plans
- Continuing education reimbursement
- Interest-free loans

Chapter 30

TERMINATIONS AND LAYOFFS

LAYOFFS AND OPTIONS

When bed capacity drops, staffing is reduced. Options for a nursing home when this happens include:

- Consult with the union to negotiate layoffs or temporary reductions in staff.
- Ask staff to voluntarily work shorter hours.
- Rotate early leave or reduce hours for all employees.
- Reduce staffing. Temporarily layoff most recent employees.
- Offer severance pay to employees.

TERMINATIONS

Employees can terminate employment voluntarily or involuntarily. Voluntary terminations are the result of finding other employment, moving, illness, or pursuing other goals. In the case of involuntary termination, agency policy and procedures are developed in order to:

- Protect the residents and assure quality care.
- Inform employees of the nature and seriousness of the problem behavior.
- Protect the home from lawsuits for improper terminations.

Steps in Developing Progressive Disciplinary Action and Termination Policies

Effective progressive disciplinary action and termination policies need to be complemented by clear job descriptions and performance appraisals. Each employee needs to understand their own job requirements and expectations. This must be in the form of a written document, which is signed and placed in the employee's personnel file. The performance appraisal evaluation provides one piece of documentation of the employee's performance of the job, as well as giving the employee and supervisor an opportunity to voice concerns and develop a corrective action plan.

Corrective action plans are written agreements that define a problem or unacceptable behavior, and outline a program to correct the problem. Problems may include, for example, being 5–10 minutes late to work, coming back late from a break, excessive absenteeism (2 or more days absent within a 30-day period), being boisterous on the floor, refusal to work, unexcused absences, smoking in nonsmoking areas, eating resident's food, accepting tips, sleeping on the job, theft, threatening/intimidating behavior, resident abuse, willful damage to the facility, falsification of resident or employee records, insubordination, absence for 2 consecutive days without reason, drinking alcohol on the job, using illegal drugs, etc.

The next step in developing the plan is to identify the seriousness of the problem behavior. Some behaviors are dangerous to the safety of residents (e.g., theft, abuse, alcohol consumption, etc.). Other behaviors are less dangerous, but create problems for the residents, the facility and/or the staff (e.g., being late to work, smoking, boisterousness, etc.). The appropriate consequence for failure to meet job expectations needs to be made explicit (e.g., attendance at a special training workshop, temporary suspension, loss in pay, or termination). The written plan includes actions to be taken by the employee, as well as the supervisor, and a date for re-evaluation.

Clear guidelines need to be made available to all employees on the conditions of termination. Critical and dangerous behaviors are conditions warranting immediate termination. Less dangerous behaviors require warnings to the employee. Repeated violations of agency policies and practices are also cause for termination.

Terminations and Layoffs

Corrective action plans are individualized for each employee, depending on the problem. They are developed any time a supervisor believes there is a problem that requires more than merely bringing the matter to the attention of the employee. Corrective action plans and termination policies require employees and supervisors to understand procedures for reporting and recording problem behaviors. To comply with personnel standards and to insure employees understand the seriousness of the problem, specific steps are followed.

1. Document in writing all incidents or infractions, including:
   - Description of incident
   - Date and time of incident
   - Name of person reporting incident
   - Exact quotes of what is said to the employee regarding the incident
   - Name of supervisor who talked to employee
   - Employee's signature
   - Supervisor's signature.
2. Give a copy of the report to the employee and place a copy in the employee's personnel file.
3. Submit a copy of the report to the administrator.

The following is an example of how progressive disciplinary action might be implemented in a nursing home. The first step is to define the specific indicators of unacceptable work performance and behavior. These must be specific, objective, and measurable whenever possible.

Secondly, unacceptable work performance and behaviors can be categorized according to severity and placed in groups of similar severity. For example, coming to work 5 minutes late can be equivalent to taking a break longer than permitted. In a greater category of severity would be refusing to listen to a supervisor, by not performing a specific task and not getting a glass of water to a resident who is thirsty and unable to obtain the water without assistance.

Point values can be assigned to each category so that minor offenses account for one point each, moderate offenses for two points, severe offenses for three points, and dangerous offenses four points, resulting in involuntary termination. Lastly, state the consequences for an employee reaching various point levels within a given period of time (e.g. 6 months or a year), and state the amount of time which must elapse (e.g. 3 months, 4 months, etc.) for all or some of the points to be removed.

More specifically, using this point system, one point might result in an oral warning, two points in a written warning, three points in a suspension for a stated time period without pay, and four points would result in an involuntary termination. If the employee (i.e., one who has not been terminated) then goes for a period of time without further offenses (e.g. 3, 6, or 12 months) one or more points would then be removed from the record.

As some of the specified offenses listed in the progressive discipline system will most likely be of a subjective nature and open to interpretation (e.g., threatening/intimidating behavior, dangerous behavior, untidy appearance, discourtesy to the public, etc.), and because extenuating circumstances can relate to what seems to be offenses of a clearly objective nature, it is important to establish a reasonable system of appeals to both protect the employee from unfair treatment and to protect the nursing home from needless lawsuits. It is advisable to consult with a competent attorney for determining reasonable procedures and time guidelines when establishing an appeals process.

APPENDICES

APPENDIX A

Resident Assessment Checklist: Admissions

The following list is to be used by all departments as a guide for items to include on a departmental assessment form for each resident. This is not an exhaustive list and is only intended to provide basic information about the resident.

General Resident Information
— name
— preferred name/nickname
— birthdate
— birthplace
— gender
— age
— admission date
— name/title of assessor
— source of assessment information
— date of assessment
— race/ethnic background
— language spoken
— marital status
— emergency contact person
— height
— weight
— room number
— names, addresses and phone numbers of family members, significant others, etc., important to resident
— religious affiliation

Legal Status
— guardianship status
— power of attorney
— responsible person

Medical Profile
— primary physician
— eye doctor
— dentist
— medical diagnosis
— resident information regarding diagnosis
— physician's informed estimate of discharge potential
— diet
— surgery history
— current medications
— type of appliances used
— continence

Admissions Form

Date _____

Assessor _____ Room # _____

Resident name _____ Facility # _____

Date admitted _____ Previous residence _____

Sources of assessment _____

Basic Information

Preferred name _____ M   F   Age _____

Born on _____ In _____

Marital status _____ Race _____

Religious affiliation _____ Spoken language _____

Education level _____ Previous occupation _____

Emergency Contact Person

Name _____ Relationship _____

Address _____ Phone _____

Legal Status

Physician _____ Address _____ Phone _____

Diagnosis(es) _____

_____ Resident informed?   Y   N

Physician's estimate of restorative potential _____

_____

Dentist _____

Eye doctor _____

Other doctor(s) _____

Surgical history _____

Current medications _____

Height _____ Weight _____ Appliances _____

APPENDIX B

Resident Assessment Checklist: Activities

Use the following list as a guide for items or categories to consider including in an Activities Assessment Form.

General Resident Information
— name
— preferred nickname
— birthdate birthplace
— gender
— age
— height
— weight
— admission date
— name/title of person doing assessment
— source of assessment information
— previous occupation
— race/ethnic background
— veteran status
— education
— marital status
— emergency contact person

Legal Information
— guardianship status
— power of attorney
— responsible person for resident

Medical Profile
— primary physician
— dentist
— eye doctor
— diagnosis
— resident informed of diagnosis
— physician's informed estimate of discharge potential
— diet
— surgical history
— appliances
— eyeglasses
— hearing aid
— continence
— prescriptions

Involvement
— community
— spiritual
— active
— sedentary

Ability to Participate in Activities Emotional/Psychological
— orientation
— social skills/participation
— personality
— psychosocial evaluation
— adjustment to nursing home and disability
— social skills
— types of activities recommended

(continued)

Reader Assessment Checklist: Activities (*continued*)

Physical Limitations
— ambulation
— hearing
— vision
— diet
— coordination
— M.D. approval for participation in activities
— types of activities recommended
— sensory stimulation
— physical activity
— adjustment to disability

Interest Inventory
— types of activities preferred
    service
    intellectual
    physical
    community
— type of interaction preferred
    individual
    one-on-one
    group

Appendix B

Activities Assessment Form

Resident _____ Room # _____ Admission date _____

Physical Limitations
Physician approval in chart for participation in Activity Program?   yes   no
Date of approval _____   Contraindications _____

L	**Arms**	R	L	**Hands**	R		**Hearing**
☐	full motion	☐	☐	full motion	☐	☐	no problems
☐	partial motion	☐	☐	partial motion	☐	☐	hearing aid
						☐	poor hearing
☐	no function	☐	☐	no function	☐	☐	deaf (r or l)
☐	paralysis	☐	☐	paralysis	☐		

Vision
- ☐ no problems
- ☐ glasses for reading
- ☐ glasses all the time
- ☐ blindness (r or l)
- ☐ needs large print books

Balance/Strength
- ☐ poor
- ☐ fair
- ☐ good

Ambulation
- ☐ independent/walk
- ☐ wheelchair
- ☐ walker/cane
- ☐ bedridden

Diet
- ☐ regular
- ☐ diabetic
- ☐ other _____
- ☐ self-feed
- ☐ needs assistance

Communication
- ☐ speaks well
- ☐ mumbles
- ☐ good comprehension
- ☐ has difficulty comprehending

Types of Activities Recommended (check all that apply)
- ☐ reality orientation
- ☐ remotivation
- ☐ entertainment
- ☐ social interaction
- ☐ arts/crafts
- ☐ spiritual/religious
- ☐ intellectual stimulation
- ☐ service to others

- ☐ sensory stimulation
- ☐ physical activity
- ☐ provide emotional expression
- ☐ community outings

Method
- ☐ one-on-one
- ☐ small group
- ☐ large group
- ☐ volunteer contact

Personality (traits and moods as observed)
- ☐ active
- ☐ cheerful
- ☐ considerate
- ☐ talkative
- ☐ unselfish
- ☐ argumentative
- ☐ complaining

- ☐ irritable
- ☐ selfish
- ☐ bored
- ☐ clinging
- ☐ gloomy
- ☐ restless
- ☐ unresponsive

- ☐ withdrawn
- ☐ self-sufficient
- ☐ patient
- ☐ other _____
  _____
  _____
  _____

Activities Assessment Form (*continued*)

Likes _____

_____

Dislikes _____

_____

Interest Inventory
Past/present **community/organizational** involvement (e.g., lodges, clubs, veterans, political, etc.)

_____

_____

Preferred **sedentary** involvement   Preferred **active** involvement

Sedentary	Active
☐ watching tv	☐ walking
☐ listening to radio/music	☐ bingo
☐ reading	☐ gardening
☐ discussion groups	☐ baking/cooking
☐ board games	☐ resident advisory council
☐ current events	☐ eating out
☐ painting	☐ adopt a friend/grandparent
☐ car rides	☐ musical instrument(s)
☐ talking on telephone	☐ shuffleboard
☐ coin/stamp collecting	☐ shopping
☐ crossword puzzles	☐ dancing
☐ letter writing	☐ chapel
☐ visiting with others	☐ Bible study
☐ sewing/handwork	☐ other _____
☐ cards	
☐ crafts	
☐ other _____	

Spiritual involvement: Church interest/affiliation _____

Denomination _____ Name of clergy _____

Religious activities _____

Assessor (name, title) _____

APPENDIX C

Resident Assessment Checklist: Dietary

Use the following list as a guide for items or categories to consider for a Dietary Assessment Form.

General Resident Information
— name
— preferred name/nickname
— birthdate
— birthplace
— gender
— age
— height
— weight
— admission date
— name/title of person doing assessment
— source of assessment information
— previous occupation
— race/ethnic background
— veteran status
— marital status
— emergency contact person
— religion/minister
— funeral home

Legal Information
— guardianship status
— power of attorney
— responsible person for resident

Medical Profile
— primary physician
— dentist eye doctor
— diagnosis
— resident informed of diagnosis
— physician's informed estimate of discharge potential
— diet
— surgical history
— appliances
— eyeglasses
— hearing aid
— continence
— prescriptions affecting dietary related functioning

Physical Assessment
— height, weight
— recent weight loss or gain
— usual weight
— chewing/swallowing ability
— choking/swallowing problem
— dentures

(continued)

Resident Assessment Checklist: Dietary (continued)

Physical Assessment (continued)
— condition of own teeth
— skin
— hearing
— vision
— bladder/bowel condition
— paralysis
— deformity of hands
— shakiness of hands
— degree of ambulation
— ability to communicate
— special eating equipment/assistance

Laboratory Tests
— date of test and result:
  sodium
  potassium
  calcium
  glucose
  total lymph count
  HGB/HCT
  HGB/AIC
  cholesterol/triglycerides
  total protein
  serum albumin
  BUN
  other

Diet History/Nutrition
— diet order
— food allergies/intolerances
— attitude regarding food
— where meals are taken
— assistance needed for eating
— percentage of food usually eaten
— supplements, vitamins/minerals
— medications affecting diet or nutrition
— medications affecting ability to eat
— daily intake: milk, juice, water, coffee/tea
— food from outside sources
— current meal intake
— excessive consumption of food/beverage
— beverage preferences
— food preferences
— typical meal: breakfast, lunch dinner
— usual meal times prior to admission

Psychological Factors
— reaction to placement or diagnosis that affects dietary intake
— resident's response to diet order
— factors involved:
  boredom
  loneliness
  anxiety
  apathy
  anger
  depression
  others

Plan of Care
— problems/needs
— possible goals
— possible approaches
— proposed reassessment date

Appendix C

Resident Assessment Form: Dietary

Date admitted _____ Name _____ Room # _____
Date assessed _____ Assessor _____ Facility # _____

Physical Assessment
Diagnosis _____ Check all that apply:
_____ ☐ Constipation
Medications affecting diet _____ ☐ Diarrhea
Height _____ Weight _____ ☐ Vision impairment
Ideal weight _____ Explain _____
Chewing: ☐ Dentures ☐ Nausea
☐ Own teeth ☐ Dehydration
☐ No teeth ☐ Hearing impairment
Condition of mouth _____ Explain _____
Swallowing ability _____ ☐ Incontinence
Skin condition _____ ☐ Other
Catheter yes no Explain _____
Decubitus or prone to breakdown? yes no
Describe _____ Describe any physical limitations _____

Psychological Factors   **Laboratory Results**
factors affecting diet: Date of tests _____
(check all that apply) Serum Albumin _____ BUN _____
☐ Boredom Total Protein _____ Glucose _____
☐ Loneliness Sodium _____ Total lymph count _____
☐ Anger Potassium _____ Hgb/hct _____
☐ Depression Calcium _____ Cholesterol _____
☐ Other Other _____

Nutrition and Diet History
Diet order _____ Food from outside sources _____
Attitude toward food/diet order ___ Assistance required _____
_____ % of food usually eaten _____
Food allergies _____ Where meals usually taken _____

Current daily intake		Likes	Dislikes
Juice ___	Supplements/	_____	_____
Milk ___	vitamin-mineral ___	_____	_____
Coffee/Tea ___		_____	_____
Typical foods eaten at		Usual meal time	Additional notes
breakfast ___	snack _____	_____	_____
lunch _____	beverage _____	_____	_____
dinner _____		_____	_____

APPENDIX D

Resident Assessment Checklist: Nursing

Use the following list as a guide for items or categories to consider including on a Facility Assessment Form.

General Resident Information
— name
— preferred name/nickname
— birthdate
— gender
— age
— admission date
— name/title of assessor
— source of assessment information
— date of assessment
— race/ethnic background
— languages spoken
— marital status
— educational background
— veteran status
— emergency contact person
— height
— weight
— vital signs
— mode of transportation
— physician's name
— skin condition
— orientation
— medical diagnosis
— discharge potential
— medical history
— surgical history
— current medication
— current diet
— rehabilitation orders
— standing orders
— social history mental assessment information

Medical Profile
— primary physician
— eye doctor
— eyeglasses
— diagnosis
— hearing aid
— continence
— prescriptions

Legal Information
— guardianship status
— power of attorney
— person responsible for resident

Pre-Admission Data
— prior living arrangements
— incidents and conditions leading to admission
— resident's involvement in placement decision

(*continued*)

Resident Assessment Checklist: Nursing (*continued*)

Physical condition
— ambulation
— locomotion
— range of motion
— specific medical conditions
    decubitus ulcer
    diabetes mellitus
    Foley catheter in place
    gastronomy
    paralysis
    sutures in place
    appliances in place
    prosthesis
    pain
    other
— vision
— hearing
— incontinence
— behavior
— reality orientation

Occupational Therapy Issues
— ability to dress self
— ability to feed self
— personal hygiene
— ability to communicate

Nursing Assessment Form

Date assessed _____ Room # _____
Assessor _____ Facility # _____

Primary MD _____ Admitted from _____
Consulting MD _____ Transported by _____
Dentist _____ Sex M F Date of birth ___ Age ___

Major Medical Diagnosis _____

Discharge Potential **Diet**
☐ Less than 50% _____
☐ Roughly 50-75% _____
☐ Greater than 75% _____

Physical Conditions
☐ Decubitus ulcers   Special diet   Pain
☐ Diabetes mellitus ☐ Low salt   Type _____
☐ Foley catheter   ☐ Diabetic   Location _____
☐ Gastrostomy   ☐ Liquid
☐ Paralysis   ☐ Low fat   Prosthesis
☐ Sutures in place   ☐ Bulk   Type _____
☐ Appliances in place

Criteria	0	1	2	3	Score
State of health	Good	Fair	Poor—declining	Serious	___
Age	< 60	60–70	70–80	> 80	___
Body	Well nourished	Obesity	Thin	Debilitated	___
Mental status	Alert	Confused	Lethargic	Comatose	___
Activity	Ambulates alone	Ambulates w/assistance	Chair only	Bedfast/bedrest	___
Mobility	Full	Restricted	Very restricted	Immobile	___
Fluid intake	Good	Fair	Poor	None	___
Predisposing diseases	Absent	Slight	Moderate	Severe	___
				Total	___

Residents with scores above 12 should be considered at risk and should be placed on a decubitus prevention plan, which includes aspects of medication, treatment, nutrition, and repositioning/massage.

Evaluation date _____ Risk score _____

Nursing Assessment Form (*continued*)

Condition of Resident's Skin
Visually indicate with code numbers the following conditions:

Body marks	Rash
1. Tattoos	8. Mild
2. Birth marks	9. Severe
3. Other _____	10. Allergic
Broken areas	Reddened area
4. Sores	11. Location
5. Grafts	Verbal description
6. Sutures	_____
7. Other _____	_____

Restorative Nursing Section

Ambulation
☐ Bedfast
☐ Stands, but does not walk
☐ Transfer, but does not walk
☐ Gait

Exercises
☐ Range of motion
☐ Passive range of motion
☐ Wheelchair exercises
☐ Independent

Bathing
☐ Bed bath
☐ Needs help into tub/shower
☐ Requires little help
☐ Independent

Vision
☐ Blind
☐ Impaired
☐ Glasses
☐ Normal 20/20

Locomotion
☐ Cannot move from place to place
☐ Requires wheelchair
☐ Must be led
☐ Independent

Dressing
☐ Must be dressed
☐ Needs a lot of help
☐ Minimal help
☐ Dresses self

Feeding
☐ Must be fed
☐ Feeds self with help
☐ Feeds self

Hearing
☐ Deaf
☐ Hard of hearing
☐ Hearing aid
☐ No problem

Grooming
☐ Needs help staying clean
☐ Needs help with clothes
☐ Needs help with hair

Incontinence/toileting
☐ Independent
☐ Needs assistance
☐ Stress related
☐ Soils occasionally
☐ Soils most of time

Speech
☐ Clear, distinct
☐ Difficult to understand
☐ Signs/gestures
☐ Non-verbal
☐ Sounds
☐ Does not respond to others
☐ Responds to signs gestures
☐ Understands others

Behavior and Reality Orientation

☐ Verbally abusive
☐ Depressed
☐ Afraid
☐ Anxious
☐ Sociable

Orientation to place
☐ Always
☐ Sometimes
☐ Never

☐ Attention
__ screaming
__ slaps
__ hits
__ pinches

Nursing Assessment Form (*continued*)

Orientation to time
☐ Always
☐ Sometimes
☐ Never

Orientation to person
☐ Always
☐ Sometimes
☐ Never

Social Assessment

Visitors
☐ Family members
_____
_____
☐ Friends
☐ Volunteers

Family is
☐ Supportive
☐ Helpful
☐ Accepting of placement

Adjustment to environment
☐ Does not like room, facility, or grounds
☐ Wants to go home
☐ Complains about everything
☐ Appears pleasant, well-adjusted

APPENDIX E

Resident Assessment Checklist: Social Services

Use the following list as a guide for items or categories to include on a social services assessment form.

General Resident Information
— name
— preferred nickname
— birthdate
— birthplace
— gender
— age
— marital status
— height
— weight
— admission date
— name/title of person doing assessment
— source of assessment data
— previous occupation
— race/ethnic background
— education
— veteran status
— emergency contact person

Legal Information
— guardianship status
— power of attorney
— responsible person for resident

Medical Profile
— primary physician
— dentist
— eye doctor
— diagnosis
— resident informed of diagnosis
— physician's informed estimate of discharge potential
— diet
— surgical history
— appliances
— eyeglasses
— hearing aid
— continence

Involvement
— community
— spiritual
— active
— sedentary

Pre-Admission Data
— prior living arrangements
— incidents and conditions leading to admission
— person responsible for resident

Personal
— habits
— likes and dislikes

Psychosocial Assessment
— memory deficits
— attention span
— awareness of environment
— orientation to time, place, and person
— consistency of orientation
— spatial awareness of body
— wandering activity
— ability to communicate
— responsiveness to others

Financial Information
— sources of resident's payment
— HMO membership number
— social security number
— medicare number
— medicaid number
— veteran's number
— S.S.I. number
— family contribution

Adjustment to Illness and/or Placement in Facility
— anxiety related to illness/aging
— fear of dying
— indications of adjustment or nonadjustment to placement
— anxiety related to finances
— attitude toward family
— family attitude toward resident
— degree of cooperation
— physical abusiveness
— verbal abusiveness
— history of suicidal attempts
— sexual problems
— depression
— involvement in group activities
— independent activities

Discharge Planning
— estimation of discharge possibilities
— community resources to facilitate discharge

Resident Assessment Form: Social Service

Date assessed _____ Resident _____ Room # _____
Date admitted _____ Facility # _____

Pre-Admission Data

Place of residence before admission   Attitude toward admission
_____   Resident _____

Reason(s) for admission   _____
_____   Family _____
_____   _____

Family and Social Information
Names, addresses, and telephone numbers of important family and friends

_____
_____
_____
_____

Church interest or affiliation
Church _____ Denomination _____ Minister, Priest, Pastor, etc. _____

Discharge Planning (check one)

almost always	some- times	almost never	
☐	☐	☐	Orientated to day/month/year
☐	☐	☐	Good attention span
☐	☐	☐	Aware of environment
☐	☐	☐	Answers questions correctly
☐	☐	☐	Recognizes family
☐	☐	☐	Recognizes staff
☐	☐	☐	Wanders
☐	☐	☐	Combative toward others
☐	☐	☐	Belligerant toward others
☐	☐	☐	Complains
☐	☐	☐	Able to communicate accurately
☐	☐	☐	Poor motivation to perform ADL
☐	☐	☐	Inappropriate sexual behavior

(*continued*)

Resident Assessment Form: Social Service (*continued*)

Recommended Intervention (check all that are appropriate)
☐ Reality orientation
☐ One-on-one counseling
☐ Family counseling
☐ Resident support group
☐ Family members support group
☐ Discharge counseling
☐ Clergy visit(s)
☐ Financial consultation
☐ Legal consultation
☐ Medical evaluation

Resident Involvement
List past/present **Community/Organizational Involvement** (e.g., lodges, clubs, veterans, political, etc.)

_____

_____

Preferred **sedentary** involvement
☐ Watching tv
☐ Listening to radio/music
☐ Reading
☐ Discussion groups
☐ Sew/handwork
☐ Visit with others
☐ Letter writing
☐ Other _____

Preferred **active** involvement
☐ Cards
☐ Walking
☐ Baking/cooking
☐ Exercise
☐ Gardening
☐ Dancing
☐ Musical instrument(s)
☐ Other _____

Preferred **religious/spiritual** involvement

_____

Personal

	Likes	Neutral	Dislikes		Likes	Neutral	Dislikes
Animals	☐	☐	☐	Solitude	☐	☐	☐
Outdoors	☐	☐	☐	Cold weather	☐	☐	☐
Sweets	☐	☐	☐	Company	☐	☐	☐
Flowers	☐	☐	☐	Shopping	☐	☐	☐
Sunshine	☐	☐	☐	Nice clothes	☐	☐	☐
Music	☐	☐	☐	Movies	☐	☐	☐
Silence	☐	☐	☐	Art	☐	☐	☐

Habits
☐ non-smoker   __ cigarettes
☐ smokes   __ cigars
   __ pipe   ☐ chews tobacco

Other likes/dislikes
_____
_____
_____

APPENDIX F

Care Plan Sections

Components of the care plan document are:

1. **Identification material about the resident, such as:**
   — name
   — physician's name
   — diagnosis
   — admission date
   — date of birth
   — religion
   — room number

2. **Statement of problems/needs**
   These are conditions contributing to a resident's inabilities to carry out required life tasks.

3. **Goals**
   These list what the resident should achieve after a certain period of time.

4. **Approaches**
   These are instructions to the caregivers on how to work with the resident toward the achievement of the goals.

5. **Designation of responsibility**
   This is a statement of which department, or person in the department, is responsible for implementing each approach within the care plan.

6. **Documentation of goal achievement**
   This involves a specific location or method of notation on the form which indicates whether or not a goal has been achieved.

7. **Signatures**
   Each person present at the care plan meeting signs an attendance sheet.

   Each department representative signs the care plan form for each resident.

APPENDIX G

Care Plan Document

Resident _____ Room # _____ Admission date _____
Diagnosis _____ Physician _____ Level of care _____

Indicate dates by each notation

Problems/Needs	Goals	Approaches

APPENDIX H

Areas and Types of Short-Term Goals

The care plan may address many areas of patient concern. Among these are:

1. Diagnoses related areas
2. Bowel and bladder
3. Rehabilitation
4. Mobility
5. Personal hygiene
6. Activities
7. Activities of daily living
8. Social functioning
9. Family relations
10. Community relations
11. Spiritual
12. Psychological functioning
13. Discharge planning
14. Weight
15. Dietary

There are several types of short-term goals:

1. **Improvement goals**—encourage a higher level of physical, psychological or social functioning.

2. **Maintenance goals**—aimed at keeping the patient at his present level of health and functioning and/or retarding the rate of severity of deterioration.

3. **Preventive goals**—aimed at preventing complications.

4. **Palliative goals**—directed at making the patient more comfortable.

5. **Coping goals**—directed at helping a patient understand, accept, and develop a positive attitude toward and/or compensate for his condition or limitation.

APPENDIX I

Care Card (front)

Resident _____   Room # _____

Approaches   Goals

— Keep side rails up at all times while   Will prevent skin
  in bed.   breakouts.
  Turn and position every 2 hrs.
  Use pillows between legs when on
  side.
— Elevate contracted leg with pillows
  when on back.

Care Card (back)

Resident _____   Room # _____

Approaches   Goals

Special Shift Tasks

7–3

3–11 Resident bath prior to bedtime.

11–7 Inform charge nurse of resident
     request for sleeping pill.

APPENDIX J

Goal Checksheet

Goal and Approach

	1	5	9	13	17	21	25	29
	2	6	10	14	18	22	26	30
	3	7	11	15	19	23	27	31
	4	8	12	16	20	24	28	32
	1	5	9	13	17	21	25	29
	2	6	10	14	18	22	26	30
	3	7	11	15	19	23	27	31
	4	8	12	16	20	24	28	32
	1	5	9	13	17	21	25	29
	2	6	10	14	18	22	26	30
	3	7	11	15	19	23	27	31
	4	8	12	16	20	24	28	32
	1	5	9	13	17	21	25	29
	2	6	10	14	18	22	26	30
	3	7	11	15	19	23	27	31
	4	8	12	16	20	24	28	32
	1	5	9	13	17	21	25	29
	2	6	10	14	18	22	26	30
	3	7	11	15	19	23	27	31
	4	8	12	16	20	24	28	32

All entries must be initialed and initials identified by full name in signature area.

Signature/Initial
(Night Shift)

Signature/Initial
(Day Shift)

Signature/Initial
(Evening Shift)

APPENDIX K

Development Flow from Diagnosis to Approach

Diagnosis   Alzheimer's Disease

Problem   Confusion
Problem affects the resident's well-being when he/she wanders from the facility building.

Need   The resident has a need to be safe within the supervised confines of the building.

Goal   Resident will wander from wing no more than 2X/week by (date).

Strengths   Excellent walking skills. Pleasant, follows verbal instructions. Readily accepts assistance and guidance.

Approaches   **Nursing:** Walk with resident to and from dining room 3X daily.
Activities: Walk with resident to activities, explain where you are and why you are there.
All staff: When resident walks near the outside door, verbally redirect towards resident's room.

APPENDIX L

Sample Job Description
Nurse's Aide 7:00 A.M.–3:30 P.M.
Qualifications

Education: A minimum of a grammar school education with a high school education or equivalent preferred. Certificate from Certified Nurse's Aide Training program preferred.

Training and Experience: Previous experience with elderly preferable.

Job Knowledge: Knowledge of procedures and techniques involved in administering simple treatments and providing related bedside care to residents. Must be familiar with the location of the various departments of the home. Understanding of standard techniques used in providing personal services for residents and in caring for equipment and supplies. Must understand the basis of good sanitation and sterile techniques to avoid infection or spread of contagious illnesses.

Working Environment: Work indoors in well-lighted and ventilated areas. May be exposed to communicable diseases. Possibility of strains due to moving residents.

Performance Requirements

Responsibility: Handling and caring for residents to ensure their safety and comfort. Adhering to instructions issued by nurse. Performing duties in accordance with the methods and techniques which conform to the home's standards of quality. Providing maximum resident care service as directed. Maintaining good housekeeping standards within assigned duty areas.

Physical Demands: Good physical and mental health. Constant standing and walking during work periods. Turning, stooping, bending, stretching, and lifting to assist residents, make beds, move equipment, and perform other related tasks. Finger and hand dexterity to handle delicate instruments and other equipment. Visual and hearing acuity to detect changes in resident's condition.

Special Demands: Must have a genuine interest in geriatric nursing. Willingness to work with the realization that errors may have serious consequences for residents. Patience and tact in dealing with residents, their families, and visitors. Some initiative and judgment in recognizing symptoms indicating a resident's adverse reactions to treatments. Willingness to perform a variety of simple repetitive tasks, many of which involve unpleasant conditions.

Job Duties

1. Set up clean and dirty linen carts daily.
2. Review your assignment of residents and their plan of care, including your cleaning assignment, break assignment, and any special instructions.
3. Receive report from the staff nurse about your residents, such as:
   a) anything that is different or special you need to do for resident
   b) any new admissions
   c) any job assignments not included in the written assignment.
4. Make rounds to check all assigned residents. Be sure residents are prepared for breakfast. Face and hands are to be washed. Oral hygiene is done, toileting or diaper change is completed, and residents are set up for breakfast in bed, chair, or dining room.
5. Pass breakfast trays, seeing that each resident receives proper diet and that the meal is hot. Set up tray for eating, butter bread, open milk carton, etc. according to resident's needs. Note how much each resident eats for documentation on patient care record and advise nurse of any decreased intake.
6. Trays of residents requiring spoon feeding or partial assistance with actual feeding shall be served last.
7. Collect all meal trays and place on diet carts. Clean overbed tables. Position residents according to turning schedule as needed and document on the turning schedule as you complete each turn.
8. Give bed baths and showers as assigned daily including shampoos and nail care. Record care done in the patient care record. Report to the nurse any bruises, cuts, scratches, rashes, or any change in the resident's skin condition.
9. See that all residents are properly dressed and that hair is combed neatly. Give priority to residents going into therapy. Apply urinary leg bags as ordered, use medical aseptic technique, cover large drainage bag tubing with a fresh sterile catheter cap, and empty the bag of urine.
10. Complete room, make beds, and see that clothing is put away and table tops and dressers are clean. Put personal soiled clothes in dirty linen cart and throw it in laundry chute by 11 A.M.
11. Place soiled diapers in plastic bags, close by knotting, and discard in garbage chute.
12. Incontinent residents are to be checked every 2 hours and changed as needed. Assist continent residents in toileting as needed.
13. Check and toilet residents on bladder training at 8 A.M., 10 A.M., noon, and 2 P.M. or according to the individual's care schedule. Document on the training schedule and the I&O sheet.
14. See that position of bedfast residents, those with restraints, and those at high risk of pressure sores is changed every 2 hours or more. Document turning schedules as each turn is completed.

Appendix L

15. Report any unusual symptoms to charge nurse such as pain, fever, body rash, personality change, or any change in the resident's condition whether physical, emotional, or psychological.
16. Pass fresh water to all residents able to take fluids by mouth. Assist and encourage residents to drink fluids frequently unless otherwise ordered.
17. Pass morning and afternoon nourishments as assigned.
18. Prepare residents for lunch. See that residents going to dining room are taken on time. Repeat procedure as for breakfast.
19. Assist residents out of dining room after meal. See that they are clean, neat, and comfortable. Assist those who require a nap to bed.
20. Any units of discharged residents are to be cleaned by housekeeping and the bed made with fresh linens by the nurse's aide assigned to that room. Pack belongings as instructed by the charge nurse.
21. Assist in ambulating residents as requested by the Rehab Department or charge nurse. Do ROM and ADL on residents assigned to you according to sheets and as requested, and complete documentation.
22. Answer call lights promptly and courteously whether or not it is your assigned resident. Answer call lights for other staff when they are on break. They will do the same for you. Keep the call light within the resident's reach.
23. Assist with admissions, including settling the resident in the room and completing vital signs and the clothing list.
24. Complete documentation on I&O, B&B, V.S., Patient Care Record, and any other forms required.
25. Be sure safety restraints are on where needed. All restraints must be released at least every 2 hours and the resident repositioned and/or ROM done as appropriate for the type of restraint used.
26. Make last rounds by 2 P.M., changing diapers, toileting, and turning residents as needed.
27. Clean off your linen carts and put them at the linen room for next shift.
28. Report to the charge nurses on the resident's condition and whether or not your assigned work was completed by 2:45 P.M.

I, _____ , have read the above job description and fully understand the conditions set forth therein, and if employed as a Nurse's Aide, I will perform these duties to the best of my knowledge and ability.

Date _____ Signature _____

APPENDIX M

Role-playing as a Problem Solving Method

At staff meetings, select employees from various departments to role-play the parts of residents and staff to find creative solutions to problems in the facility.

Example

The nursing home is having a problem with Mrs. Evans, an 88-year-old blind resident who complains of hunger even after meals. She complains by yelling very loudly. The only solution to the problem so far has been to wheel her into her private room so that the other residents and staff are not disturbed by the noise.

A dietary aide is selected to play the part of Mrs. Evans. He sits in a wheelchair and yells that he is hungry, just as he has heard Mrs. Evans do. A nurse's aide is selected to try to solve the problem as the other staff members watch.

First, the aide tries to reason with Mrs. Evans. She tells the resident that she cannot possibly be hungry since she has just completed dinner and even left food on her plate. Mrs. Evans continues to yell. The aide decides to wheel Mrs. Evans from the hallway, where she is parked in her chair, to her room. Mrs. Evans yells even louder when the aide tells her she is taking her to her room. The aide decides to wheel Mrs. Evans to a location near the nurses' station. She tells Mrs. Evans that she must be quiet so that the nurses' important work is not disturbed. The dietary aide playing Mrs. Evans pretends to be curious about what the nurses at the desk are saying so he (she) stops yelling in order to listen.

The staff watching the "play" decide to try parking Mrs. Evans near the desk during the day to see if she will be so interested in listening to the nurses' activity that she will no longer cause a disturbance by yelling.

The solution is tried for several days. The nurses and aides working at the desk pay some extra attention to Mrs. Evans as they work by saying hello as they pass by and complimenting her on her appearance. Mrs. Evans, who was a very lonely and unhappy resident, enjoys listening to the activity she cannot see, and she enjoys the companionship of the nurses and aides as they work. She no longer complains or yells and the problem is solved.

APPENDIX N

Sample Minutes from a Staff Meeting

Minutes: Utilization Review Meeting 6-15-92

Present: Shirley Campbell (Administrator), Dr. Philip Ramsey (Medical Director), Deborah Parsons (DON), Jerry Thorsen (SSD), Carol Simon (Activity Dir.), Maude Butler (Dietary Supervisor), Rick Baxter (Maintenance Supervisor)
Recording Secretary: Deborah Parsons
Starting time: 10:00 A.M.
Ending time: 11:30 A.M.

I. Announcements
- Next scheduled meeting: 10-14-92, 10:00–11:30 A.M.
- Welcome to Carol, our new activity director!
- Census: 123 residents (Medicaid-52, Private-71)

II. Old Business
A. Decubitus Ulcers:
- At last meeting (2-13-92) there were five cases.
- As of date (6-15-92) there are three cases.
- What has been done: An in-service was held 2 months ago by the DON for all aides. Discussion was held on the conditions surrounding decubitus ulcers and a new rotation schedule was presented. The new schedule was implemented by the aides on all three shifts. A follow-up in-service was held 1 week later to discuss how the new program was working.
- What will be done: Due to positive feedback from the aides using the schedule and the decrease in decubitus cases, the program will continue to be used.

III. New Business
A. Medication Combinations:
- Dr. Ramsey gave a presentation on medication combinations that can be harmful to residents with certain diagnoses.
- As of yet there have been no incidents of conflicting combinations in the facility; we would like to maintain our awareness.

B. Resident Involvement in Care Plan Meeting:
   - Jerry (SSD) presented a questionnaire he designed to be completed by residents on attending their own care plan meeting.
   - After reviewing the questionnaire, staff present voted on whether the survey should be distributed. Voting resulted in: 6 Yes, 1 No.
   - Jerry will make arrangements to distribute the questionnaire.

Meeting Adjourned

APPENDIX O

Examples of Suggestions from the Employees' Suggestion Box

- Put non-skid mats or appliques in residents' bathtubs.
- Use linen tableclothes instead of plastic for holiday or special meals.
- Have reserved employee parking.
- Give employees their birthdays off as paid holidays.
- Install a juice machine in the employees' lounge.
- Replace artificial plants with live plants.
- Have an employee "best attendance" award periodically.
- Replace harsh soap in dispensers with a milder soap.

APPENDIX P

Sample Job Evaluation of Nurse's Aide

	Almost Always	Usually	Adequate	Seldom	Never
Appearance and Conduct					
— uniform neat and clean, dresses neatly, good body hygiene	☐	☐	☐	☐	☐
— cooperates with peers	☐	☐	☐	☐	☐
— cooperates with supervisors	☐	☐	☐	☐	☐
— accepts correction and is willing to improve	☐	☐	☐	☐	☐
— completes assigned tasks	☐	☐	☐	☐	☐
— enthusiastic toward resident care	☐	☐	☐	☐	☐
— respects resident's privacy	☐	☐	☐	☐	☐
— interacts appropriately with residents' significant others	☐	☐	☐	☐	☐
Dependability					
— reports to work on time	☐	☐	☐	☐	☐
— reports to work per schedule	☐	☐	☐	☐	☐
— assignments are followed through on a timely basis	☐	☐	☐	☐	☐
Quality of Care					
— resident rooms and work areas kept clean and neat	☐	☐	☐	☐	☐
— attends to residents' needs (feeding & elimination)	☐	☐	☐	☐	☐
— grooms residents appropriately (teeth brushed, shaved, hands and face washed and clean)	☐	☐	☐	☐	☐

	Almost Always	Usually	Adequate	Seldom	Never
Quality of Care (*continued*)					
— interacts in a polite way with the residents	☐	☐	☐	☐	☐
Safety					
— safely handles equipment used (wheelchairs locked during transfer, restraints on, etc.)	☐	☐	☐	☐	☐
— consistently uses infection control (hand washing, linen care, etc.)	☐	☐	☐	☐	☐
— keeps cabinets and doors locked (snackroom, storage, supplies, etc.)	☐	☐	☐	☐	☐
— corrects or reports unsafe conditions	☐	☐	☐	☐	☐
Documentation and Execution					
— records daily charting	☐	☐	☐	☐	☐
— carries out programs per care plan objectives	☐	☐	☐	☐	☐
Other Items					
— attends staff meetings and in-services regularly	☐	☐	☐	☐	☐
— ability to establish working relationship with fellow employees and residents' significant others	☐	☐	☐	☐	☐

Overall Evaluation

___ Outstanding
___ Very Good
___ Satisfactory
___ Needs Improvement
___ Unsatisfactory

Comments

Comment on employee's major strengths, developments achieved since the last appraisal.

If overall evaluation is "Needs Improvement" or "Unsatisfactory," list steps employee is to undertake to continue employment.

Employee's comments on appraisal:

Prepared by (supervisor's signature) _____

Approved by (Administrator or DON) _____

This appraisal was discussed with me
(employee's signature) _____ Date _____

APPENDIX Q

Sample Newspaper Article Topics

- Announcements of residents' birthdays
- "Someone You Should Know" articles about residents
- Upcoming craft shows presented by staff and residents
- Awards to outstanding staff members
- Resident-family activities or programs
- Talks given by residents
- Fund-raisers for the nursing home
- "Why I Love My Grandparents" writing contest for children
- A person from the community spends a day as a resident and reports on the experience
- Publish residents' poetry or short stories

APPENDIX R

Example of a Letter to Family Members

Dear _____

One of the most important goals of our nursing home is to strive to create a facility environment in which families can feel comfortable expressing concern and loving support for family members.

As family members, you can be valuable contributors to the well-being of your loved one, and to the facility in general. On the following page, please indicate the ways you would like to be involved. You will be notified of the dates and times of the events and programs in which you are interested.

Thank you for your involvement. We look forward to serving you in policies and programs that enrich the quality of family relationships, the lives of the residents, and the nursing home as a whole.

Sincerely,

Family of (resident's name) _____ Date _____

Please place a check beside the activities in which you are interested in participating:

Resident Care Plans
- ☐ I would like to be notified of **every** care plan meeting involving my relative so that I may attend.
- ☐ I would like to be notified **periodically** of care plan meetings involving my relative so that I may attend.
- ☐ I would like to be notified only of major problems or concerns regarding my relative.
- ☐ I would like to be notified only in case of emergencies regarding my relative.

Family Programs
- ☐ I am interested in attending a community support group to help family members make difficult decisions and to cope effectively with their concerns.

☐ I am interested in attending workshops that can enrich communication and visiting skills with my relative as well as help in understanding the aging process.

I am interested in attending the following family activities:
☐ monthly coffee houses with staff and other families
☐ resident/staff/family holiday parties
☐ community outings for residents and families
☐ family committees on facility policies

APPENDIX S

STANDARDS OF QUALITY ASSURANCE

As the long-term care field continues to grow, increased attention is given to standards and measurements of quality assurance. Current federal guidelines require a quality assurance program be in place at each long-term care facility. Many professional organizations have established standards of practice for their particular discipline. The most commonly recognized and used standards are those of the Joint Commission on Accreditation of Healthcare Organizations for long-term care facilities. It is beyond the scope of this volume to list all the standards for each area within the nursing home. Instead, a list of some of the organizations which may be contacted for further materials on standards of practice is provided.

Sources of Information

American Association of Homes for the Aging
1050 17th Street, N.W.
Washington, DC 20036
(202) 296-5960

American College of Health Care Administrators
8120 Woodmont Ave., Suite 200
Bethesda, MD 20814
(301) 652-8384

American Congress of Rehabilitation Medicine
30 N. Michigan Ave.
Chicago, IL 60602
(312) 236-9512

American Health Care Association
1200 75th St., NW
Washington, DC 20005
(202) 833-2050

American Hospital Association
840 N. Lake Shore Dr.
Chicago, IL. 60611
(312) 280-6382

American Medical Association
535 N. Dearborn St.
Chicago, IL 60610
(312) 944-2722

American Nurses Association
2420 Pershing Road
Kansas City, MO 64108
(816) 474-5620

American Psychiatric Association
1700 18th, N.W.
Washington, DC 20009
(202) 797-4900

Campaign for Quality Care
1424 16th St., N.W., Suite 12
Washington, DC 20036
(202) 797-0647

Center for the Study of Aging and Human Development
706 Madison Ave.
Albany, NY 12208
(518) 465-6927

Health Care Financing Administration
Office of Survey and Certification
Division of Long Term Care Services
Meadows East Building, Area 2-D2
6325 Security Blvd.
Baltimore, MD 21202
(410) 966-6784

Appendix S

Joint Commission on Accreditation of Healthcare Organizations
875 North Michigan Ave.
Chicago, IL 60611
(312) 642-6061

National Association of Social Workers
7981 Eastern Ave.
Silver Spring, MD 20910
(301) 565-0333

National Council on Aging
600 Maryland, S.W., #100
Washington, DC 20024
(202) 479-1200

National Council of Senior Citizens
925 15th St., NW
Washington, DC 20005
(262) 347-8800

National Geriatrics Society
212 W. Wisconsin Ave. Third Floor
Milwaukee, Wisconsin 53203
(414) 272-4130

National Hospice Organization
1901 North Fort Myer Dr., Suite 920
Arlington, VA 22209
(703) 243-5900

National Rehabilitation Association
633 South Washington St.
Alexandria, VA 22314
(703) 836-0850

Veterans Administration
810 Vermont Ave., NW
Washington, DC 20420
(202) 389-3781

Additional information can be received from local Medicaid, Medicare, and Social Security Administration offices.

REFERENCES

Abrahams, R., & Lamb, S. (1988). Developing reliable assessment in case-managed geriatric long term care programs. *Quality Review Bulletin, 14*(6), 179–186.

Alan, L. (1984). The importance of including the family in the comprehensive psychiatric assessment of the nursing home bound person. *Journal of Gerontological Social Work, 7*(3).

Alexander, G.P. (1985). Monetary rewards can bolster productivity." *Contemporary Long Term Care, 8*(7), 39–40.

Alfaro, R. (1986). *Application of nursing process: A step-by-step guide.* Philadelphia, J.B. Lippincott Company.

Bainum, R. (1985). Bonus incentives can promote image and care. *American Health Care Association Journal, 11*(3).

Bowman, M. (1986). Peer level leaders spark higher job performance. *Provider, 12*(3), 44–45.

Buckholdt, D.R. (1983). The family conference. *Journal of Family Issues, 4*(4), 613–631.

Caldwell, J.M. (1980). Managing patient care under the new standards. *Contemporary Administrator, 3*(12), 6–8.

Christopher, A., & Meunier, G.F. (1986). How gaming can solve your attendance problem." *Nursing Homes, 1,* 31–33.

Committee on Nursing Home Regulation, Institute of Medicine. *Improving the quality of care in nursing homes.* Washington, D.C.: National Academy Press.

Cox, C., & Ephross, P.H. (1989). Group work with families of nursing home residents: Its socialization and therapeutic functions. *Journal of Gerontological Social Work, 13*(3–4), 61–73.

Crawford, S.A., Waxman, H.M., & Carner, E.A. (1983). Using research to plan nurse aide training. *American Health Association Journal, 9(1)*, 103–104.

Day, J.M., & Berman, H.J. (Eds.). (1989). *Successful nurse aide management in nursing homes.* Phoenix: Oryx Press.

DiBerardinis, J., & Gitlin, D. (1980). A holistic assessment model for identifying quality care indicators in long-term care. *Long Term Care and Health Services Administration, 4(3)*, 227–235.

Elbert, N.F., & Smith, H.L. (1982). Inservice education and the nursing home administration. *American Health Care Association Journal, Volume B,* 30–34.

Flood, A., & Scott, R. (1987). *Hospital structure and performance.* Baltimore: John Hopkins University Press.

Getzel, J. (1982). Resident councils and social action. *Journal of Gerontological Social Work, 5(1–2)*, 179–185.

Gray, J.W. (1979). Patient care planning: A format for easy implementation. *American Health Care Association Journal, 5(3)*, 12–16.

Gray, J.W., & Aldred, H. (1980, Nov.). Care plans in long-term facilities. *American Journal of Nursing,* 2054–2057.

Greenbloot, C.T. (1984). A cure for many ills. *Contemporary Administrator for Long Term Care, 7(8),* 38–42.

Gubrium, J.F. (1980). Doing care plans for long term care. *Social Science and Medicine, 14(A),* 659–667.

Gubrium, J.F. (1980). Patient exclusion in geriatric staffings. *The Sociological Quarterly, 21,* 335–347.

Halburn, B.T., & Fears N. (1986). Nursing personnel turnover rates over potential positive effects on resident outcomes in nursing homes. *The Gerontologist, 26(1),* 70–76.

Hammond, D.R. (1986). Skillful evaluation can bring effective staff performance. *Provider, 12(5),* 45.

Hatch, R., & Franken, M. (1984). Concerns of children with parents in nursing homes. *Journal of Gerontological Social Work. 7(3).*

Hinkley, N.E. (1986). Training assures the edge on competition. *Provider, 12(3),* 28–32.

Hopping, B. (1976). Conversations in the waiting room for death. *Nursing Homes, 25(6),* 12–16.

Hughes, M., & Roller, M.E. (1986). *Social service care plans for nursing homes.* Houston, Texas: M & H Publishing Co.

Hunt, J.M., & Maran, D.J.M. (1986). *Nursing care plans: The nursing process.* (2nd. ed.). New York, New York: John Wiley & Sons.

Jeffries, B. (1986). Are you managing at peak performance? *Provider, 12(3),* 9–13.

Kane, R. (1981, Oct.). Assuring quality of care and quality of life in long-term care. *Quality Review Bulletin.*

Kleinknecht, M.K., & Hefferin, E.A. (1982, July/August). Assisting nurses toward professional growth: A career development model. *The Journal of Nursing Administration*, 30-36.

Komaroff, A. (1985). Quality assurance in 1984. *Medical Care, 23(5)*.

Kooperman, L., Schoenhofer, S., & Pyner, J. (Eds.). (1988). *Nursing home management: A people-oriented perspective*. Springfield, Illinois: Thomas.

Kraft, M.R. (1985). Quality assurance in 1984. *Medical Care, 23(5)*.

Linn, M., & Gurel, L. (1982, Fall). Family attitude in nursing home placement. *The Gerontologist*, Part 1.

Locke, M. (1987). *Revised practical guide to health care planning for nurses in long term care*. Houston, Texas: M & H Publishing Co.

Lowe, M.A. (1986, August). Care plans help manage patients as individuals. *Provider*, 48-49.

Mayers, M.G. (1983). *A systematic approach to the nursing care plan*. (3rd. ed.). Norwalk, Connecticut: Appleton-Century-Crofts.

McMurray, J., (Ed.). (1990). *Creative arts with older people*. New York: Haworth Press.

Montgomery, R. (1983). Staff-family relations and institutional care policies. *Journal of Gerontological Social Work, 6(1)*.

Morrow-Winn, G. (1983, March/April). Staff development is more management than training. *Nursing Homes*, 6–11.

Neil, M.C., Cohen, P.F., Cooper, P.G., & Reighley, J. (1985). *Nursing care planning guides for long-term care*. (2nd. ed.). Baltimore, Maryland: Williams & Wilkins.

O'Drisscoll, D. (1976). The nursing process and long-term care. *Journal of Gerontological Nursing, 2*(3), 34–37.

Patchner, M.A. (1989). Permanent assignment: A better recipe for the staffing of aides. In J.M. Day & H.J. Berman, *Successful nurse aide management in nursing homes*. Phoenix: Oryx Press.

Puckett, R.P. (1983). Corrective action: A tool for effective performance. *Contemporary Administrator, 6*(11), 25–28.

Robertson, R.D. (1988). Recreation and the institutionalized elderly: Conceptualization of the free choice and intervention continuums. *Activities, Adaptation and Aging, 11*(1), 61–73.

Sancier, B. (1984). A model for linking families to their institutionalized relatives. *Social Work, 29*(1), 63–65.

Sander, P. (1986). *Activity care plans for long term care facilities*. Houston, Texas: M & H Publishing Co.

Savishinsky, J. (1985). Pets and family relationships among nursing home residents. *Marriage and Family Review, 8*(3–4), 109–134.

Schlossberg, A. (1981, January/February). Self appraisal. *Nursing Homes*, 2–9.

Schwartzben, S.H. (1989). The 10th floor family support group: A descriptive model of the use of a multi-family group in a home for the aged. *Social Work with Groups, 12*(1), 41–54.

Scott, R., & Flood, A. (1985, Winter). Costs and quality of hospital care: A review of the literature. *Medical Care Review, 41*, 213–261.

Silvermarie, S. (1988). Poetry therapy with frail elderly in a nursing home. *Journal of Poetry Therapy, 2*(2), 72–83.

Smith, H.L., & Elbert, N.F. (1979). Evaluating employee performance. *American Health Care Association Journal, 5*(2), 10–16.

Sorodo, K. (1982). Group family counseling: An aid to long-term care. *Journal of Long Term Care Administration, 10*(1), 137–142.

Stove, V. (1974). Patient care assessment: A managerial strategy. *Journal of Long Term Care Administration, 2*(4), 18–24.

Stryker, R. (1982). The effect of managerial intervention on high personnel turnover in nursing homes. *Journal of Long Term Care Administration, 10*(3), 21–33.

Thurman, A.H., & Piggins, C.A. (Eds.). (1982). *Drama activities with older adults: A handbook for leaders.* New York: Haworth Press.

Vandenbosch, T.M., Bentley, C.L., Desiree, B., & Jones, K.A. (1986). Tayloring care plans to nursing diagnoses. *American Journal of Nursing, 86*(3), 313–314.

Wagnild, G., & Manning, R.W. (1986). The high turn-over profile: Screening and selecting applicants for nurse's aide. *Journal of Long Term Care Administration, 14*(2), 2–4.

Walton, K. (1987). *Writing health care plans: A handbook for food service supervisors.* Houston, Texas: M & H Publishing Co.

Ware, P.J. (1980). Multidisciplinary care. *Nursing Homes, 29*(3), 21–24.

Williams, C. (1986). Improving care in nursing homes using community advocacy. *Social Science and Medicine, 23*(12), 1297–1303.

INDEX

Accountability, structuring of, 104–106
Active relationship, in management, 104
Activities, resident assessment checklist for, 175–178
Admission(s)
  learning about resident before, 7–8
  resident assessment checklist for, 173–174
Advertising, for staff, 111–115
Affirmative Action, 111, 125
Aide documentation, 41, 152
Anniversary, employment, 162
Annual nurses recognition day/week, 162
Appearance, in performance appraisal of aide, 151
Applications, staff, distributing and receiving of, 117–119
Applicants
  initial screening of, 119
  screened, interviewing of, 119–124
Appraisal, see Performance appraisal(s)
Approach(es), 33–52
  development of, 33–34
  diagnosis to, development flow from, 196

listing of, 34
management, 101–106
responsibility for, 34–35
staff, 4
Assessment
  of applicant, by interviewer, 122
  of home's goals and objectives, 155
  of in-service training needs, 156, 167–168
  resident, see Resident assessment entries
Assignment, permanent, to residents, 41
Assignment of responsibility
  for approaches, 4, 34–35
  for assessment, 8
Assurance, 57
Authority, structuring of, 103–104

Behavioral goals, 31–32
Benefits
  employee, 165–166
  of quality assurance, to families, 73–77

Care, quality of, see Quality of care
Care card(s), 38–39, 194

Care plan
  communication of, to staff, 28, 37–41
  fine-tuning of, 42
Care plan document, 192
  sections of, 191
Care plan meeting, 19–28, 52
  adjournment of, 28
  and communication of care plan to direct care providers, 28
  delegation of duties among team members in, 24–25
  designation of coordinator for, 24
  development of care plan in, 26–27
  discussion of resident's problems, needs and strengths in, 26
  evaluation of goals in, 25–26
  interdisciplinary team for, 23
  involvement of residents and family members in, 23–24
  productive setting for, 20–21
  recording of information on care plan form in, 27
  repetition of previous steps in, 28
  schedule for, development of, 21–23
Care planning, 1–53
  process of, 3–4
Certification programs, 112
Certified Nurse's Aide (CNA), 112
Charge nurse, job description for, 138–140
Client of nursing home, recruitment of family as, 75
Collecting information, 9–10
Communication of care plan, 28, 37–41
Community image, positive, quality assurance and, 69–71
Competent performance, 144
Conduct, in performance appraisal of aide, 151
Confidentiality, of employee records, 126–127
Consulting relationship, in management, 104
Coordinator, care plan, 24
Cost effectiveness, quality assurance and, 83–85

Definition of standards of excellence, in cost-effectiveness, 85
Delegating responsibility, 103–104
Delivery, fine-tuning and monitoring of, 42
Dependability, in performance appraisal of aide, 151
Development, of staff, *see* Training and development
Diagnosis(es)
  to approach, development flow from, 196
  and goals, 30
Diagnosis-linked problems, 14
Dietary concerns, resident assessment checklist for, 179–181
Direct care providers, communication of care plan to, 28, 37–41
Discharge potential, and goals, 30
Disciplinary action, 168–170
Document, care plan, 192
Documentation, 43–46, 53
  accessibility of, to staff, 46
  aide, 41, 152
  consistent format in, 44–45
  daily, 45
  of goal achievement status, 49
  periodic summaries in, 45
  requirement of, 44
Duties, description and performance of, in job analysis questionnaire, 131

Educational background
  in job description, 134, 138, 197
  of staff, 107
Employee benefits, 165–166; *see also* Staff
Employee of the month, 162
Employees' suggestion box, 203
Employment anniversary, 162
Environment
  quality assurance and improvement of, 79–81
  working, *see* Working environment
Equal Employment Opportunity, 111, 125

INDEX

Evaluation, *see also* Performance appraisal(s)
  in cost-effectiveness, 85
  of effectiveness of approaches and goals, 25–26, 47–50, 53
  of family quality assurance program, 77
  of in-service training, 160
  job, of nurse's aide, 204–205
  quality assurance and, 57, 89, 92, 94, 95
Example, setting of, by management, 102–103

Family members
  benefits of quality assurance to, 73–77
  involvement of, in care plan meeting, 23–24
  letter to, 207–208
Fine-tuning care plan, 42
Formal quality assurance programs, 89–91, 92–94
Functional problems, 14–15

Goal achievement status, 48–49
Goal checksheet, 39–41, 195
Goal performance, data about, 47–48
Goals
  management, in training, 158–159
  and objectives, assessment of, 155
  resident, *see* Resident goals

Health Care Financing Administration, 11
Hiring, of staff, 117–124
Household income, of staff, 108

Identification of needs, *see also* Definition of standards
  of families, 75, 77
  for individual safety, 79–80
  quality assurance and, 57, 88, 89, 92, 93, 95
  of residents, 4, 10, 13–16, 17, 26
Illinois Department of Public Aid, 32
Image, positive community, quality assurance and, 69–71

Implementation, 37–42, 52
  in cost-effectiveness, 85
  of family quality assurance program, 77
  of performance appraisal, 149
  quality assurance and, 57, 89, 92, 94, 95
Incentive plans, 161–164
Income, household, of staff, 108
Informal quality assurance programs, 91–92, 93, 94–95
Information
  collecting of, 9–10
  recording of, on care plan form, 27
  shared during interview, 122–123
Informing each department, of new resident, 8
In-services, for staff, 162
In-service training
  assessment of needs for, 156, 157–158
  conducting of, 159–160
Inspections of facility, in training, 156
Institutionalization, 30
Insurance, employee, 165
Interdisciplinary team, 23
Internal announcements, in recruiting staff, 115
Interpersonal recognition and incentives, 162
Interviewing screened applicants, 119–124
Intuitive judgments, in staff interview, 122

Job analysis, 129–133
Job description, 129, 134–140
Job duties
  for charge nurse, 138–140
  for nurse's aide, 135–137, 198–199
Job evaluation, of nurse's aide, 204–205
Job knowledge
  for charge nurse, 138
  for nurse's aide, 134, 197
Job posting, 113–114

Lake Bluff Health Care Center, 157
Language, spoken, of staff, 108

Layoffs, staff, 167
Leadership styles, 24–25
Learning about resident, before admission, 7–8
Letter, to family members, 207–208
Life, quality of, mission of, 59–62
Longevity, employee, 165

Management
 personnel, 99–170
 quality assurance and, 63–67
Management approach, 101–106
Management goals, in training, 158–159
Management problems, 15–16
Measurable goals, 31–32
Medicaid, 11
Medical problems, 14–15
Medicare, 11
Merit pay plan, 141, 142–145
Minimum Data Set (MDS), 11–12
Mission, quality of life, 59–62
Monitoring delivery, 42
Morale, staff, 161–164

Needs
 identification of, see Identification of needs
 in-service training, assessment of, 156, 167–168
 resident, 4, 10, 13–16, 17, 26
Newspaper advertisements, in recruiting staff, 114, 115
Newspaper article topics, 206
Nurse's aide(s)
 documentation by, 41, 152
 interview questions to, 121
 job description for, 134–137, 197–199
 job evaluation of, 204–205
 orientation skills checklist for, 157
 performance appraisal of, 151–152
Nursing, resident assessment checklist for, 182–186
Nursing home
 environment of, see Environment
 goals of, see Goals

Organizational chart, 105
Organizational incentives and recognition, 162–164
Orientation, staff, 155–156, 157
 benefits of, 153–154
Outstanding performance, 144
Overlapping shifts, 42

Parties, staff, 161–162
Peer appraisals, 149
Performance, see also Merit pay plan
 of duties, in job analysis questionnaire, 131
 goal, evaluation of, 47–48
Performance appraisal(s), 147–152; see also Evaluation
 of aide, 151–152
 benefits of, 147–148
 components of, 148–149
 implementation of, 149
 steps in conducting supervisory, 150
 in training, 156
Performance requirements, in job description
 for charge nurse, 138
 for nurse's aide, 134–135, 197–198
Permanent assignment, 41
Personnel management, 99–170; see also Staff entries
Personnel records, 125–127
Physical demands, in job description
 for charge nurse, 138
 for nurse's aide, 134, 197
Physical effort, in job analysis questionnaire, 132
Plan(s)
 care, see Care plan entries
 incentive, 161–164
Planning
 care, 1–53
 in cost-effectiveness, 85
 for family needs, 75–77
 quality assurance and, 57, 89, 92, 94, 95
Positive community image, quality assurance and, 69–71

Problems
  resident, 4, 10, 13–16, 17, 26
  solving of, see Solving problems
Psychosocial problems, 15

Qualifications, in job description
  for charge nurse, 138
  for nurse's aide, 134, 197
Quality, 57
Quality assurance, 55–97
  attainment of, 87–97
  benefits to families of, 73–77
  cost effectiveness of, 83–85
  management and staff and, 63–67
  nature of, 57–58
  and nursing home environment, 79–81
  positive community image of, 69–71
  and quality care, 59–62
  standards of, 209–211
Quality assurance program(s), 89–95
  development of, 95–97
  formal, 89–91, 92–94
  informal, 91–92, 93, 94–95
Quality of care
  in performance appraisal of aide, 151
  quality assurance and, 59–62
Quality of life mission, 59–62

Realistic goals, 31–32
Reassessment, periodic, 10
Recognition
  interpersonal, 162
  organizational, 162–164
  structured, 161–162
Recording, of information, on care plan form, 27
Records, personnel, 125–127
Recruitment
  of family, as client of nursing home, 75
  of staff, 111–115
Reference checks, 123, 124
Registration reimbursement, 160
Rehabilitation, 30
Reimbursement, for training, 160

Relationships, consulting and active, in management, 104
Resident(s)
  informing each department of new, 8
  involvement of, in care plan meeting, 23–24
  learning about, before admission, 7–8
  problems, needs, and strengths of, 4, 10, 13–17, 26
Resident appraisals, 149
Resident assessment, 5–12, 51
  assigning responsibility for, 8
Resident assessment checklist
  for activities, 175–178
  for admissions, 173–174
  for dietary concerns, 179–181
  for nursing, 182–186
  for social services, 187–190
Resident Assessment Instrument (RAI), 11
Resident goals, 4, 29–32, 52
  areas and types of short-term, 193
  evaluation of, in care plan meeting, 25–26
Responsibility
  for approaches, 4, 34–35
  for assessment, 8
  delegating of, 103–104
  in job analysis questionnaire, 133
  in job description, 134, 138, 197
Retired Seniors Volunteer Program (RSVP), 71
Role-playing, as problem solving method, 200
Rounds, 105–106
  in training, 156

Safety, in performance appraisal of aide, 151–152
Safety needs, individual, identification of, 79–80
Salaries, 141–142
Satisfactory performance, 144
Scheduling, of in-service training, 159–160

Scholarship/tuition reimbursement, 160
Screened applicants, interviewing of, 119–124
Screening, of applicants, initial, 119
Self appraisal, 149
Service options, 165
Setting example, by management, 102–103
Sex, of staff, 108–109
Shifts, overlapping, 42
Skills, in job analysis questionnaire, 132
Skills checklist, 157
Social services, resident assessment checklist for, 187–190
Solving problems; *see also* Implementation; Planning
 quality assurance and, 88
 role-playing and, 200
Special demands, in job description
 for charge nurse, 138
 for nurse's aide, 134–135, 198
Spoken language, of staff, 108
Staff, *see also* Employee *entries*; Job *entries*; Personnel *entries*
 accessibility of documentation to, 46
 advertising and recruitment of, 111–115
 communication of care plan to, 28, 37–41
 composition and retention of, 107–109
 documentation requirement for, 44
 hiring of, 117–124
 merit pay plan for, 141, 142–145
 performance appraisal of, 147–152
 quality assurance and, 63–67
 salaries of, 141–142
 terminations and layoffs of, 167–170
 training and development of, 153–160
Staff approaches, 4
Staff meeting(s)
 sample minutes from, 201–202
 in training, 158
Staff morale, 161–164
Standards, of quality assurance, 209–211
State mandated in-services, 158
Stating values, 101–102
Strengths, resident, 4, 10, 13–14, 16–17, 26
Structured incentives, 161–162
Structuring
 of accountability, 104–106
 of authority, 103–104
Subordinate appraisals, 149
Suggestion box, employees', 203
Supervisory appraisals, 149
 steps in conducting, 150
Support, innovative, to staff, 41–42

Team, interdisciplinary, 23
Team members, delegation of duties among, 24–25
Terminal care institutionalization, 30
Terminations, staff, 167–170
Training and development, 153–160
 benefits of, 153–154
Training and development program
 development of, 155–160
 elements of, 154–155
Training and experience, in job description
 for charge nurse, 138
 for nurse's aide, 134, 197

Unsatisfactory performance, 144

Values, stating of, 101–102
Volunteers, and cost effectiveness, 84

Word of mouth, in recruiting staff, 112
Working conditions, in job analysis questionnaire, 133
Working environment, in job description
 for charge nurse, 138
 for nurse's aide, 134, 197